ANCIENT WISDOM

Distributed by
P & R Medical Services, Inc.
P.O. Box 262488
Plano, TX 75026
www.AncientTravels.com

ISBN-13: 978-1508885207
ISBN-10: 1508885206

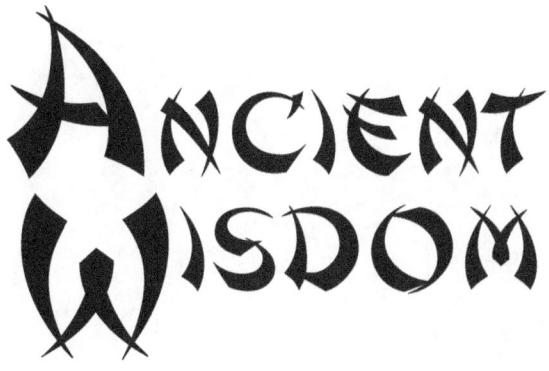

ANCIENT WISDOM

A Further Continuation of a Discourse Between a Master
and His Student on Acupuncture and Chinese Martial Arts

Richard A. Peck, L.Ac.

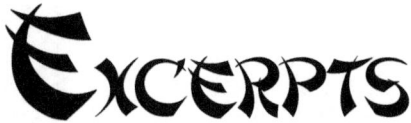Excerpts

"When you look at the twenty-four hour energy clock, there are certain times when energy is at its maximum."

"One way to treat this problem is to insert needles around the area where the patient has the pain."

"We use the acupuncture point Feng Long which is four inches below Tsu San Li for treating mucus and chest congestion."

"Master, while we wait, will you share with me more information about Tai Chi Chuan, Pa Kua Chang, and Hsing-Yi Chuan?"

"Each one of the elements in Hsing-Yi Chuan has more than one application."

"The liver is a Yin organ and its complimentary opposite as you know is the gall bladder, which is Yang."

"You are not the first person to ask about the function of one point on a meridian in relation to other points on the same meridian."

"Master, you have mentioned that we are a system of energy and as such we are part of an overall system of energy. In other words, if I understand what you have told me in the past, we are a system within a system."

"It is a misconception held by both individuals and doctors that we are a composite of unrelated systems and, therefore, a composite of unrelated illnesses."

PREFACE

This is the third novel explaining Traditional Chinese Medicine (TCM), Chinese internal martial arts, and Chinese culture. The first novel published in late 2009 introduced basic concepts of TCM and some fundamentals of Chinese internal martial arts.

The second novel published in 2013 enhanced material introduced in the first novel and put forth some intermediate concepts of TCM and Chinese internal martial arts.

This, the third novel, explores some advanced concepts of TCM and Chinese internal martial arts. The characters, setting, plot, and writing style of this novel are consistent with the first two novels. As with the other two books, this is an instructional novel. Rather than present the material all at one time, the approach of using a novel as a teaching tool was well accepted. In the process of elaborating on TCM and martial arts, it continues narrating the fictional travels of Liu Bin and his student Pei Ke as they journey through northern China.

Hopefully, this novel, like the previous two, will educate the reader in an entertaining way on the complexity and richness of this ancient medicine.

Readers of *Ancient Travels* and *Ancient Knowledge*, were kind enough to give me constructive suggestions for this sequel. Those who enjoyed reading about martial arts wanted an expansion of the theories of Tai Chi Chuan,

Pa Kua Chang, and Hsing-Yi Chuan. Others were happy with the Chinese martial arts, but wanted additional and expanded concepts of TCM. These comments were instrumental in the continuation of the travels of Liu Bin and Pei Ke.

My gratitude goes to my teachers Huo Chi Kwang, Lu Hung Bin, Dr. Ineon Moon, and Dr. Tsao Cheng Chang for sharing with me information they might not have shared with others. I feel blessed that they went out of their way to insure I understood the information they wanted me to learn.

Once again, I want to thank my wife, Iva Lim Peck for taking time out of her busy schedule to read the initial manuscript and make sure there are no blatant TCM errors. As in the first two novels, I am using one of her Chinese paintings for the cover of the book. Jen Sin Lau of Singapore once again used her knowledge of classical Chinese to provide the Chinese translation of the title to this book. I want to thank Jerry Robinson and Dave Pinkard for reading the initial manuscript. Their suggestions enhanced the readability of the story.

Many thanks also go to Landa Miller for reading the manuscript and making appropriate corrections. Her comments and suggestions have made the manuscript more readable and enjoyable. She was also kind enough to write a commentary, which I have used for the back cover of the book.

Once again, I asked Mat Rayback to do the final edit of the manuscript, and prepare the book for printing. Mat has a wonderful way of taking my rough manuscript and turning it into a finished readable product.

To the many students and patients I have had over the last thirty years who unknowingly taught me so much about how to be both a good practitioner of TCM and a better teacher of martial arts I offer my sincere thanks.

As I mentioned in the previous two books, this novel is strictly a work of fiction. While there may appear to be names and places familiar or similar, there is no similarity between the characters mentioned in this book or the other two books to any individuals past or present.

I have tried to accurately describe, in some detail, the geographic locations in China, the concepts of TCM, and the concepts of Chinese internal martial arts. Any errors or omissions in this work are strictly of my own doing.

Hopefully, you will enjoy this book like you did the first and second novels. I was pleased to learn that as a result of reading the first two novels, many readers have expressed an interest in using TCM for their health care needs and in studying one or more of the Chinese internal martial arts.

For those of you who have read the first two books, I hope the information has provided you with the knowledge you need to ask appropriate questions when you find a practitioner of TCM or teacher of Chinese internal martial arts. Very often, we accept information presented to us without questioning the validity of that information. Understanding the fundamentals and concepts of TCM and Chinese martial arts will go a long way in having a positive outcome in your treatments or studies.

If you have any suggestions or comments, I do value your opinion and would enjoy hearing from you.

Richard A. Peck, L.Ac. (June 2015)
www.AncientTravels.com
www.IntegratedCenterForOrientalMedicine.com
info@ICFOM.com

CHAPTER 1

Liu Bin and his protégé Pei Ke finished their lengthy conversation with Sun Han, and were in the process of leaving when Liu turned to Sun.

"Sun, I don't like asking, but I need a favor from you."

"I am indebted to you for saving my life," said Sun Han. "If it is feasible, I will do it."

"Pei Ke and I need two fast sturdy horses, but I have no way to pay for them."

As soon as he asked his question, Liu felt a shift in the Universal Energy and for the first time Pei Ke felt it too. It was a sensation of deep foreboding unlike anything he'd felt before. He looked at Liu in alarm and immediately knew that his master had felt the same thing. They needed to go soon. Lives depended on their immediate departure.

After arrangements were made about the horses, Liu Bin and Pei Ke left Sun Han's office and wasted no time in returning to where they had been staying. They retrieved their meager belongings.

"Pei Ke, do you have everything including my sack and the amulet?" asked Liu.

"Yes, Master. I have everything."

They stepped out the doorway, turned left, and walked quickly down the street. After a few steps, Liu looked back at the door one final time and wondered when he would return. Half a block later, Liu abruptly stopped and turned to Pei Ke.

"Pei Ke, do you think you can find your way to the corral by yourself?"

"Yes, Master. The directions Sun Han gave us were very clear. Where are you going?"

"I must make one or two stops before leaving Beijing. It won't take me very long."

"Master, let me come with you. What if you need help?"

"I am fine. Now do as I ask and go quickly. I will not be too long, and I will meet you and Sun Han at the north gate of the corral. Now go."

Pei Ke turned and quickly walked down the street, following the directions given by Sun Han. He felt nervous and alone. During their time in Beijing, there had only been a few times when he hadn't been with his teacher. Of course, on those days when he was not with his teacher, he wondered what Liu Bin was doing, but it would have been inappropriate for him to ask. After all, it was Liu who had brought him to Beijing, not the other way around.

He wondered now if Liu's business had anything to do with Chen Chang. Briefly, he considered following Liu in case he needed help, but ruefully decided to do what he was told. There was always a logical reason for Liu Bin's actions and besides, Pei Ke wasn't sure what he could do to help anyway. More likely, he'd get in the way.

Walking down the street, he felt the same uneasiness that had descended on him in Sun Han's office. It was like a void, like energy was being sucked out of him, but when he looked around, he couldn't see anything unusual. There were people walking up and down both sides of the street. There were a couple of men over by one of the vegetable stalls looking his way but he didn't feel that was too unusual or out of place. Maybe he was experiencing what Liu had experienced more than one time. Was Liu still feeling it? He quickened his pace to distance himself from the area, and to find the corral as quickly as possible.

When Pei Ke was out of sight, Liu turned in the opposite direction and hurriedly walked down the narrow street. He needed to see two people before leaving. No matter how important it was to leave quickly for his ancestral home, this was just as important. Leaving Beijing again without saying goodbye would be unthinkable. He had made a terrible mistake years ago, and he was not going to make it again. This time there was more at stake. Hopefully, he would be able to find who he was looking for without too much trouble.

Walking quickly through the narrow streets of Beijing, Liu sensed he was again followed by an evil type of energy and the energy was close. The eyes that had been following him for the last few months were again on the hunt, and to distract himself from their mystery, he wondered if Pei Ke had progressed enough in his ability to tap into the Universal Energy to sense it as well. He could not focus on such speculation for long, however, and so he turned his thoughts to Sun Han and some of the discussions they had.

Liu had known Sun for many years, since the days when he was in Beijing studying. They had met one day in one of the many teahouses and became close friends. Sun now worked in one of the offices of the emperor. Usually an office was inside the Forbidden City, but this was one instance where an official office was purposely located outside the walls of the emperor's residence.

Imperial edicts prohibited outsiders from entering the Forbidden City without an invitation. There had to be a way for the emperor to conduct the country's business without everyone entering into the royal area. Sun was one of the appointed officials outside of the gates, who conducted daily business for the emperor.

Even though he was an official of the imperial court, he did not report directly to the emperor. He reported to one of the eunuchs, who in turn reported to another eunuch. Sun was not sure how many levels of eunuchs there were, and he really didn't care. He did his job and he did it well. He went out of his way to make sure his decisions were in keeping with the wishes and sometimes whims of the emperor. He often wondered if the emperor really knew what happened outside the high walls where he was in residence. He suspected many times that the emperor really did not run the daily activities of the country; rather the eunuchs made the daily decisions. He was sure some of these decisions were more for the benefit of the eunuchs then the emperor.

For this reason and other reasons, he disliked the eunuchs. They had a certain false sense of importance, which they went out of their way to communicate to everyone. He understood they were there in part to make sure the emperor's harem did not get disturbed, but he felt there were very capable men who were not eunuchs who could do just as well.

There was some speculation on Sun's part when Liu, years earlier, abruptly departed Beijing. Liu came to his house to say goodbye. That was the last Sun saw of Liu for many years until he showed up at Sun's office that day.

Sun listened to the story Liu told him. Liu explained how Liu's family, who Sun had never met, had been killed by Chen Su and how Liu had taken revenge on the attackers, killing them all except for Chen Chang who had escaped. He related how he and Pei Ke were attacked numerous times while traveling to Beijing. Liu knew the attacks, as well as the murder of his family, were due to the land his father and grandfather before him owned.

Liu asked Sun Han to look at the document, which his grandfather received many years earlier, delineating the ownership of the land. Liu asked Sun to verify that this was indeed the Liu's family land, and he had rightful ownership to the land. Liu produced a document given to him by his father.

After close examination, Sun indicated the document Liu possessed gave full and legal ownership of the land to the Liu family. The emperor's seal and wording was in keeping with the way the emperor gave lands to loyal subjects. As far as Sun was concerned, from his careful examination, there were no discrepancies in the document, the wording of the document, or the imprint of the seal on the scroll.

Liu was pleased to hear what had been in his family for so many years, was in reality still in his family; and there were no other legitimate outside claims to the land as far as he knew. However, Liu was quite upset to find out from Sun that Chen Su's son, Chen Chang, who had escaped Liu's wrath, had actually been at Sun's office only a couple of days earlier, and presented a document purportedly giving to the Chen family the land that Liu's parents had occupied and claimed.

Sun assured Liu that the document, the Chen family had received, was given to the Chen family by a local warlord, who had conscripted individuals to fight for him in the name of the emperor. It was not an official document from the emperor himself. In essence, the document Chen had was only as good as the importance of the warlord.

In this instance, Sun had heard that this specific warlord had been killed in one of the regional battles; therefore, the document giving the land to the Chen family would be valid only if there was no other document superseding it. In this case, Liu's document took precedence over Chen's document not only because of the earlier date on the document, but also because the document came from the emperor, thus giving the Liu family the sole rightful ownership of the land.

Sun went on to explain to Liu that if there were no other members of the Liu family to contest the claim of Chen, and there was no other document besides the one Chen had in his hand then the emperor might be willing to acknowledge that Chen's document had some merit. Sun also explained that even though the Liu family had ownership of the land through the benevolence of the emperor, all lands in the empire actually belonged to the emperor and his family. The emperor could take back the land at any time; however, the likelihood of this happening was quite remote.

Liu instantly realized Hua Yee, his niece, was in eminent danger from Chen Chang. All Chen had to do was to eliminate Hua Yee and her siblings and then kill him. Chen could then claim the land for himself.

Liu explained to Sun Han the precarious situation his niece Hua Yee was in and the need to immediately return to his ancestral home. Chen Chang and his men were on horseback and he and Pei Ke did not have any means of returning to his ancestral village unless they walked and that would take too long. Time was of the essence. Sun told them to go to the emperor's corral, which was located outside of the Forbidden City, and he would meet them there.

It was in this corral, that the emperor kept not only his best horses, but also horses the imperial guards considered past their prime, and were being sold off to buy new horses. It was these good but marginal horses, Sun Han was going to sell in the name of the emperor to Liu and Pei Ke for their journey back to Liu's ancestral home.

CHAPTER 2

Pei Ke arrived at the north gate of the corral and immediately the caretaker greeted him with suspicion.

"Can I help you," he said.

Sun Han had told them that he knew the caretaker of this stable well and had many dealings with him, so Pei Ke answered confidently.

"I am waiting for Sun Han. I spoke with him earlier today. He will be here shortly."

It was unclear if the man believed him or not. His expression didn't change.

"You must wait outside the corral, away from the horses," he said.

Wondering why the caretaker was so grouchy, Pei Ke walked around the corral and looked at the horses. According to Sun, this corral was but one of many stables the emperor owned. Pei Ke was amazed that a person could own so many horses. It was truly a sign of his wealth. Ordinary people couldn't afford even one horse. Most were lucky to have an ox to help work the land.

Pei Ke continued walking the perimeter of the stables, becoming nervous when neither Liu nor Han appeared. He could see the caretaker watching his every move. He finally decided to go looking for Liu when his master arrived calmly. He didn't explain what he'd been doing or where he'd been. Pei Ke did not ask. They waited in silence for Sun Han's arrival.

"Master Liu," Sun Han said when he finally arrived. "I am sorry I took so much time. I'm afraid that my schedule is not my own. I work at the whims of those to whom I report."

Liu nodded.

"I do not expect you to get in trouble in order to help us. We are in your debt."

"Master," Pei Ke said suddenly, pretending he didn't notice Liu's stern look. "I think we're being followed. When we left Sun's office, I noticed two men outside the building. I didn't think much about it, but I think I see those same men down the road and they are on horseback."

Liu and Sun turned to look down the road. Sure enough, there were two men on horseback. They were too far away to be recognized, but were conspicuous by the fact that they were just sitting on their horses gazing in the direction of the corral.

Liu wondered why he had not sensed someone was following them. He had sensed the evil energy in the area, but not the presence of these two men. It was a sign that he was letting his own thoughts get in the way of his ability to perceive the Universal Energy. In the past, he had relied on this energy to help him in difficult times. He chastised himself for his mental lapse.

He really needed to focus. Lives depended on his actions or inactions and he needed to make sure that what he did was correct. There was little or no room for error.

"We will just have to keep an eye on them," he said, turning back to look at the stable. "There is nothing we can do now."

"Yes," said Sun. "Now if both of you will wait here, I need to talk privately with the corral keeper."

"He wasn't very nice," Pei Ke said. Both older men looked hard at him and he wished he hadn't spoken.

"He is a friend of mine," Sun said. "We've known each other for many years, but he is a little suspicious sometimes." He looked at Pei Ke. "He is responsible for buying and selling horses for the emperor. It is a heavy responsibility. As such, I think I had better talk to him alone. Do you have any money on you?"

Liu looked at Pei Ke and nodded.

"We have a little," said Pei Ke. "But not much."

"Give me a few coins, maybe two or three at the most."

"How much do the horses cost?" asked Pei Ke.

For a brief moment, Sun Han didn't answer. He just looked at Pei Ke.

"I am going to negotiate the price right now," he said finally, with a glance at Liu. "Two coins will be plenty. These horses are the ones the emperor is trying to sell. If you were to buy the best horses, the price would be more than you could afford. These horses are good horses, but they're past their prime. They will get you where you want to go, but they're just not good enough for battle. I don't think you will be in a battle, do you?"

Pei Ke thought of the many fights they had been in since they had left the temple so long ago, but he didn't say anything. He just shot a glance at Liu, who wasn't looking at him, and then reached into his pants and felt for the coins in his pocket. He picked out two and handed them to Sun Han.

He noticed as he handed over the coins that the two men on horseback were watching intently. He could feel their gaze as Sun went over to the corral keeper. They spoke quietly to each other and after a few minutes Sun handed over something to the corral keeper. Discreetly, Sun added some extra coins from his own pocket, though no one saw it.

The corral keeper pointed to two horses. Sun shook his head and pointed to two others. Pei Ke couldn't tell the difference between the two sets, but Liu could. The corral keeper wanted to give them the worst horses he had in the corral, but Sun would have no part of it.

There was a discussion and an agreement. Liu watched as the corral keeper brought the two horses to the corral gate. They were not the best horses, but they'd make the journey. In Liu's opinion, his friend had done well.

The corral keeper turned away after giving the horses to Sun, but Liu could tell that something was still being discussed. The corral keeper shook his head, but Sun said something else and the man stood there for a minute. Finally, he turned and walked toward the barn. Sun motioned for Liu and Pei Ke to come to the horses.

"They aren't the best horses," said Sun. "However, they will be good enough to get you where you are going. The stable master has graciously agreed to give each of you a saddle. They were used by the emperor's soldiers and may not be in the best possible condition, but they're functional. He also agreed to give each of you two water-filled leather flasks."

As Sun was talking with Liu, the corral keeper brought two saddles from the barn and saddled the two horses for them. Pei Ke looked at the animals and wondered if he was going to be able to do this.

"Master," said Pei Ke. "I've never ridden a horse before. I don't know the first thing to do. Have you ever ridden a horse?"

"Yes, I used to ride when I was a young man. My father insisted that all his children be proficient with a horse. But don't worry. There is a first time for everyone. Now we need to go. The corral keeper will help you to get on the horse."

Liu put his foot into the stirrups and swung himself onto the saddle. It was as Liu had expected. The horse was well trained and did not move. It stood there patiently, waiting for Liu to give the command. Liu watched as Pei Ke hesitantly got on his own horse with the help of the corral keeper. Liu said goodbye to Sun and edged the horse forward. Pei Ke's horse just stood there.

Sun turned to the corral keeper.

"Are there any imperial guards here today?"

"There are always some imperial guards here," said the corral keeper. "They come to exchange horses. However, they take their time. Most do not want to return to their duties. As a favor to them, I let them loiter around for a while. There is always good tea available and they know they can help themselves. Occasionally I have one or two of them run errands for me. Is there something you need from the guards?"

Sun thought for a second before speaking.

"Is it possible for you to have a couple of guards detain the two men on horseback up the road. Those men have been following us. I don't think they can do us any harm, but I am worried about my two friends and I think these strangers mean to cause some trouble for them. Maybe the guards can question them for a couple of hours so my friends can get a decent head start."

"Yes, I can do that," said the corral keeper. "Is there anything else I can do for you?"

"No," said Sun Han. "You have done well. I will mention your cooperation to my superiors."

Chapter 3

Riding away from the corral, Pei Ke gritted his teeth as he held on tightly to the reins of his horse. He focused on getting the horse to move. He did not see Liu looking back at the two men in the distance.

Liu knew that sooner rather than later, he would have to deal with them. With the men now behind him and Chen somewhere in front, he might get trapped into a corner and not be able to fight his way out. Either way, Pei Ke was going to get the chance to prove himself as a martial artist.

"Master," called Pei Ke. "Please wait for me. I'm having trouble getting the horse to move faster. What do I need to do to make him move?"

"Pei Ke if you want the horse to go forward, gently nudge his flanks with both feet and he will move forward. If you want him to stop, gently pull back on the reins. You have to get used to the horse and the horse has to get used to you. You will get the hang of it shortly. Just do not abuse the horse, or it may throw you."

Liu turned around, and waited for Pei Ke to catch up. From his vantage point, he saw Pei Ke struggling to get the horse to move faster. More importantly, he saw the two men in the distance. Again, he felt uneasy as he looked at them. He now felt those evil eyes watching him, waiting for him to do something. He felt they were biding their time waiting for the right opportunity.

Pei Ke finally managed to get his horse moving forward and together, they began to ride from the stables. When they had ridden another couple hundred feet, Liu turned to see what had happened to the two strangers. They started following them and Liu tensed slightly, but he relaxed when, approaching the stable four imperial guards rode out to greet the two men.

The guards pointed toward the barn and the two men on horseback pointed in Liu's direction. After a few minutes, the guards led the two men off toward the barn and Liu smiled. Sun Han must have arranged for the men to be detained. Someday he would return to Beijing to repay the favor.

"Master, how many days do we have to ride to get back to your village?" Pei Ke said. "And do you think these horses will make it all the way? I'm not a very good judge of horses, but the horses that the men have who are behind us seem to be in much better shape than these."

"It will take as many days as it takes to get there," said Liu. "I figure we should cut the travel time by a third or maybe in half with the horses. Of course, we will not be staying for very long at any one place, except to rest for the evening. Hopefully, we can stay at some of the same places we stayed at when we came this way a few weeks ago.

"I am very concerned for Hua Yee and Mr. Wu. We now know that Chen Chang intends to make claim to my parents' land, and the only way he is going to get it is if there is no one around to object to it. I do not know how he is going to do it, but I am sure that Hua Yee and Wu are both in substantial danger. If Chen Chang is willing to eliminate my family, he will have no qualms in eliminating Hua Yee and Wu.

"We should have visited Sun Han when we first arrived in Beijing. I was too caught-up in visiting with the hospital and other things. Of course, if I had visited with Sun Han when we first arrived, I would not have known that Chen Chang had gone to see him. The Universal Energy has charted the path for us and we just have to follow it. We can't change what has happened, but we can chart our future from an enlightened point of view."

CHAPTER 4

Liu calculated that Sun Han would be able to detain the two men for the better part of the day. This would give them a solid day's lead. He was sure these two were part of the group associated with Chen Chang and he wanted to avoid any confrontation as a long as he could. He hoped there were only two of them back there.

With the horses, they made good time. Liu decided to take the same road they'd used on their original journey. There were two roads they could take, but he chose the one that was a little more difficult and not quite as straight forward because, he wanted places to stay for the night. He and Pei Ke had befriended many people during their journey to Beijing, and he was sure these people would be willing to once more give them food and shelter.

After a few hours, Pei Ke felt less agitated and was getting accustom and comfortable riding a horse. He couldn't believe he was actually able to do it. He'd often wanted to ride, but had never had the opportunity to do so. A little tug to the left on the reins and the horse turned left; a tug to the right and the horse started to go right. He started to understand what Liu had said. He needed to get used to the horse and the horse needed to get used to him. He wondered how fast the horse could run with him on it. He didn't plan on trying it anytime soon, but he wondered if he'd get the chance to run the horse at a full gallop.

He settled into the saddle. He knew their mission was urgent and dangerous, but it was nice to be back on the road. He'd learned a lot in Beijing, but he'd found that he missed the time travelling with his master. He affectionately patted the horse on the neck and it shook its head slightly, acknowledging the burgeoning connection between them.

CHAPTER 5

After leaving the stable, Liu and Pei Ke continued retracing their original journey from his ancestral home. They rode past the fortune teller's shop they had visited on the way to Beijing. It looked closed and even deserted. Liu wondered if Chen's men had revisited the shop.

Late in the afternoon, just before the sun descended below the horizon, they rounded a bend in the narrow road. A farmhouse came into view not more than a hundred feet from the road. Liu nodded for them to approach. Long shadows cast on the ground as they drew near. A faint light showed through one of the small windows.

Almost as soon as they left the main road, dogs somewhere within the farmhouse excitedly announced their presence. As they approached the door, it opened and a man stood in the doorway. He was tall and burly and stood defiantly. After a few words however, the farmer realized they were no threat, and agreed to let them stay for the night.

Liu and Pei Ke needed a rest not only for themselves, but for their horses. Liu knew there was just so much an animal could withstand before it totally gave out. He had to balance his immediate desire to get back home as soon as possible with what the horses would be able to endure. He would give them a rest with water and feed and start again early in the morning.

The farmer put Pei Ke and Liu up in a small room at the rear of the farmhouse. Their quarters consisted of two beds, a desk, and a chair. A small wood stove would keep them warm under the wool blankets that lay on the bed. They took dinner with the farmer and his family. They were quiet people and did not pry into why Liu and Pei Ke were on the road. After dinner, Liu and Pei Ke retired to their room.

"Master, may I ask you some questions. I know you're preoccupied with getting back to see Hua Yee, but this question has been on my mind for a while. Are you too tired to answer questions?"

"Pei Ke, ask the question."

"Master, you have explained in detail about the concepts of Yin and Yang, Five Element Theory, and the philosophy of acupuncture. In our various conversations over these many months, you have also mentioned we are both a system of energy, and a system of energy within a system of energy. I understand the words, but to be honest, I don't fully understand the meaning behind the words. I have a vague idea of what you mean when you've talked about these systems of energy, but would you elaborate on this for me one more time?"

Liu nodded slightly before answering.

"It is a misconception held by both individuals and doctors that we are a composite of unrelated systems and therefore a composite of unrelated illnesses. For example, the air we breathe does not just fill up our lungs. The ancients discovered that our lungs are intricately related to our other organs. The same is true of our other organs, and the energy associated with each of these organs, as well.

"Continuing with my example, when we have lung issues, we need to understand the complex relationship existing between the organs if we want to understand the underlying reason for that issue, and to be able to treat the whole person and not just the symptoms. There are many doctors who simply treat the lung symptoms. Doing so may be initially beneficial to the patient as it temporarily relieves one or more problems, but in reality, it does not solve the underlying cause of the problem, and so those lung symptoms or other seemingly unrelated symptoms will manifest themselves.

"Let me say it in a different way. If you know the lung system, and how it works, and ignore other systems of the body interfacing with the lungs, then you have done the patient a disservice. In addition, if you only treat the lung system, then the patient may feel better, but the underlying issue has not gone away and may return again with the same symptoms or return with a whole other set of symptoms, both in that system or another system of the body.

"To understand what I am talking about you need to have an in-depth understanding of the concepts you mentioned: Yin and Yang, Five Element Theory, Qi, and treatment protocols."

"Yes, Master. That's what I want to know. I have all this information in my head, but I feel like it's not connected. If it were connected, then I would have a better understanding of what you're doing when you treat people, and why you're doing it. As it is now, I watch you and absorb the information. If I were to treat a patient who had the same set of circumstances and symptoms, then I would use the same points you used.

"If there was a situation where the symptoms were somewhat similar, but not exactly the same, then I might question if it would be appropriate to use the protocol I saw you use. Also, in my limited experience, I've noticed my tendency to want to use specific points for generalized problems. For example, I want to use Lieh Chue to treat all lung problems, even though I know that I probably should not. Do you see my problem?"

"Pei Ke, your questions are the same questions that have been asked by every dedicated practitioner of this art. It is an indication that you want to understand why you are doing something rather than simply following a set pattern or prescription of points. This is the difference between a master acupuncturist, who has the patient's best interest at heart, and an acupuncturist who just wants to get by. There are many who just want to get by. They are satisfied with mediocre results. Unfortunately, when a patient sees any results, even mediocre ones, they are encouraged and so continue with the mediocre practitioner, not knowing that they can get far better results with someone who has sought for answers to the kinds of questions you are asking now.

"Now, to answer your questions, we need to look at them from more than one view point. First, let's look at Yin Yang theory. You are now conversant with this theory and its complimentary opposites. Am I correct?"

"Yes, Master," said Pei Ke. "You previously explained that they are opposites like up and down, male and female, and hot and cold; and that there are numerous other complimentary opposites, especially in Chinese medicine. I also understand that there are different stages in a disease process. The disease can be in its Yin stage, which would be different from that same disease in its Yang stage. Each stage has a unique set of symptoms and requires a unique way of differentiation and treatment."

"Good," said Liu. "I want you to keep what you now know firmly in mind, but now think of Yin and Yang as a plank of wood balanced in the middle. One end is Yin and the other is Yang. When they are balanced, the plank of wood is level. If there is an excess on one end, then that end will move out of horizontal balance. If one end moves either up or down, then the other end will move in the opposite direction. Thus, as Yin increases, Yang decreases, and as Yang increases, Yin decreases."

"I understand, Master, but can you give me some examples of how this applies in medicine?"

"Everyone agrees that a body is very complex, and that because of its complexity and the interactions among its various parts we cannot make categorical statements. So, what I am going to say next may happen and it may not happen.

"When you look at the twenty-four hour energy clock, you will see that there are certain times when energy is at its maximum. Lung energy is at its maximum between one and three in the morning. When lung energy is at its maximum, you can see from the twenty-four hour energy clock that urinary bladder energy is at its minimum; and when urinary bladder energy is at its maximum between one and three in the afternoon the lung energy is at its minimum. If I were to feel the pulses at three in the afternoon, and found that the lung energy was in excess, I would question the patient about symptoms related to his lungs."

"How much excess does it have to be for me to consider it a problem?" asked Pei Ke.

"Again, think of Yin and Yang as a plank of wood balanced in the middle, level with the ground. Each one of us has a different size plank in width and length, and each one of our planks can be higher or lower to the ground. If you have a wide and long plank then you have strong Yin and Yang energy. If your plank is high off the ground then you may have a large reservoir of Yin and Yang energy, but you may be susceptible to wide swings in your Yin and Yang energy as it changes compared to those whose planks are just barely off the ground."

"Master, does this explain why some people get sick and others do not when both are exposed to the same disease process?"

"It may, but there may be other factors you need to take into consideration that might also be part of the disease process. Remember, the human body is a complex structure with different interactions continually affecting multiple parts.

"Here is a good example of Yin and Yang organs affecting each other. The liver is a Yin organ and its complimentary opposite, as you know, is the gall bladder, which is a Yang organ. In Chinese medicine over consumption of alcohol adversely affects the liver causing the possibility of a liver deficiency. Ancient acupuncturists discovered that liver energy affects gall bladder energy because of its complimentary actions of Yin and Yang. If liver energy is deficient then gall bladder energy can become excess. Gall bladder energy affects muscles and tendons when it is excess, making them tight.

"Muscles and tendons when they become tight, especially around the neck area, can cause a headache. So, you can see the liver system has an effect on the gall bladder system. This is an example of the relationship between Yin and Yang. There are many other similar relationships we will explore in the future."

"Master, what are some other relationships with liver and gall bladder energy?"

"Do you remember when we treated Mrs. Wang?"

"Yes, Master. Her diagnosis was Liver Fire Rising."

"Do you remember all the symptoms she had?"

Pei Ke thought for a moment before answering. He knew most of them and could not believe he was starting to forget things.

"Master, she was depressed, angry, and had headaches."

"Yes, you are correct. Do you think her liver energy was excess or deficient based just on what you already know?"

"Since the liver energy rose upwards, I'd guess that her liver energy was excess."

"Pei Ke, do not guess. Use your knowledge to come up with a logical answer. Did she also complain of tight muscles?"

"Master, I don't remember."

"Well, she did complain of that symptom, so here we have a situation where the liver energy is excess causing the gall bladder energy to be deficient. This is just the opposite of what we explained about alcohol affecting the gall bladder. So, we need to remember excess and deficiency can have similar symptoms; however, they are treated differently.

"Now that you understand Yin and Yang a little better, you can appreciate the complexity of the interactions between Yin and Yang. When there are complex health care issues with a patient, there are many interactions taking place. Thus, we have multiple Yin and Yang imbalances in the body."

"Master, is that why some people complain of multiple health problems?"

"Yes. As there is an increase in the various couplings of Yin and Yang, the complexity of a diagnosis increases. This is especially true of people putting off treatment for extended periods of time.

"To make the problem even more difficult to diagnose, the body is divided into Yin and Yang as a system. The left side is Yang and the right side is Yin. The upper half is Yang and the lower half is Yin. The inside is Yin and the outside is Yang. One side of our body could have a Yin problem and the other side could have a Yang problem. It is the expertise of the practitioner, which comes into play here, to ascertain the imbalances and determine how to treat the patient."

"Master, I think I need some time to think about what you've said, but could you elaborate more on my first question about energy within energy? Then I'll not ask anymore. We're both tired."

"Yes," said Liu.

"Master, if I understand what you've said, we are a system of energy, and as such, are part of a bigger, more comprehensive system of energy. I understand the words, but I'm not sure I understand the deeper significance of the concepts. Is there another way to explain these concepts from a different point of view? I mean, if I compare what I have already learned, it seems that you are saying that there are different types of energy, which implies that there are even more systems, and maybe even other different systems within those systems. Maybe I'm reading too much into all this, but then again, I'm afraid I'm not reading enough into it."

Liu smiled.

"You are not the only one who struggles to understand the concept of the Universal Energy. Many people have tried to understand this concept and just as many if not more have tried to explain it. The problem is that it is the overall concept that you have to understand. There are many instances where the pieces of the overall concept of the Universal Energy may appear to be contradictory and this contradiction poses a problem for the overall understanding of the concept."

"So, it is the Universal Energy that you have mentioned so many times before."

"Yes and no," said Liu.

Pei Ke wondered how Liu was going to explain both a yes and a no at the same time. He thought that he had a rudimentary grasp on what Liu had taught him over the last couple of years, so he couldn't decide whether this to be something new or if it was going to be a further elaboration of what he had already taught him, but on a more esoteric scale?

Liu thought for a few minutes before he answered. He had explained energy to Pei Ke more than once and each time, he'd tried to answer based on what he perceived was Pei Ke's ability to understand. He again wanted to make the answer simple, but he did not want the simplicity of the answer to diminish the content of the material.

Should he explain it in bits and pieces, and in contradictory concepts as he had originally learned it, or should he explain it as he now knew it to be through his own experience, over many decades?

"Pei Ke, from our conversations these last months and the questions you have asked me, I believe you have a good grasp of what I have already explained to you in the past. Now I am going to tell you basically, the same thing, and you may feel I am just repeating myself. Pay attention to the answer, even if it seems to contradict what you have already learned. I am going to build on what you already know and hopefully take you to the next level of understanding of what energy is and how we, as humans, interact with this energy."

Liu again paused and Pei Ke waited. He knew from past experience that he shouldn't say anything. As he waited, he thought of the way his understanding of the Universal Energy had changed over time. Yes, his understanding in the beginning was quite rudimentary, but now he was at the point where he needed to be able to feel the meaning behind the words, rather than simply regurgitate what had been explained to him in the past.

"Pei Ke, let me give you a series of examples, and from the examples you can get a more complex and higher level understanding of what is meant by the Universal Energy and the fact that we are a system of energy.

"As I have explained to you more than once, the Qi or energy that flows through us came about from our parents and grandparents. It originated from the coalescence of the energy that came about from the swirling of Yin and Yang at the beginning of time. If you look at the ancient Tai Chi symbol, you can readily see a positive and a negative factor-the white being the positive and the black being the negative. As this positive and negative swirling of energy coalesced at the beginning of time, it formed the great Yin Yang of the Tai Chi. Everything sprang from this concept of Tai Chi. Even Tai Chi Chuan, the martial art developed by Chang San Fung, can be thought of as in embodiment of the flow of energy from the original Tai Chi.

"Here is where it may be a little difficult for you to understand, so I want you to listen carefully. When a man and a woman get married, each has their own set of unique energies. Thus, each woman has her own unique Qi. However, it is not a different Qi since all Qi is the same; it is only a unique manifestation of the Qi. Since there are millions of different women, we have millions of different representations of female Qi.

"The same goes for males. There are millions of different representations of male Qi. This brings up the question of the difference between male and female Qi. Again, it is all the same Qi, only represented in its own unique way.

"The process of conception is a bringing together of the male and female representations of that unique Qi of those males and females. This is why we, basically, look the same as a species, although we each have our unique characteristics. Do you understand what I mean by this first system of energy?"

"Yes, Master. You've explained it to me before, though not in so much detail."

"Just as there is a system of Qi for us humans, there is also a system of Qi for all living things. Thus, an apple, a dog, a cat, an elephant each has within its body a representation of Qi as it relates to its species. As I mentioned, and want you to understand, this is all the same Qi, just represented differently. If it weren't for this Qi, we would not be alive.

"If we take different varieties of apples and look at them, we can see certain characteristics of each apple. One may be greener or redder than another variety, but in essence they are both apples. The Qi of each variety of apple has its own unique characteristics. Now, let's take the same variety of apple but grown in different areas of the country. Each may taste slightly different, though they have the same Qi.

"So what makes the difference between two apples that are of the same variety? It is the Qi of the soil that makes the difference. The difference could also be the amount of water the tree gets or the amount of sunlight.

"So what is the difference between the two soils? One type of soil may be subjected to more animal droppings than another. The water may be different, as we all know that some water tastes better than other water. Thus, we have different aspects of Qi in water from different areas of the country. There are many different factors, and they can be subdivided many times into smaller and smaller categories.

"So how does this Qi in our bodies work? The Qi flows in a circular pattern. I have mentioned before that it flows from one meridian to another. Since we have various organs in our bodies, we have Qi flowing within each organ. Thus, the Qi of the lung has its own representation of Qi, just as the Qi of the large intestine has its own representation. However, it is all the same Qi. And when there is something wrong with the flow or it is not balanced, we are subjected to health problems. That is where Traditional Chinese Medicine comes into play, to solve the imbalance and put the body back into harmony with itself.

"Here is another example for you to consider. You and I both have Qi or the Universal Energy. There are millions and millions of people just like us who also have Qi. Think of each of us as a drop of water in a container. If I add another drop of water, it mixes with all the other millions of drops of water. However, if I add a drop of dirty water into the container, it will in some small measure affect all the other drops of water.

"The same applies to our bodies. The Universal Energy flows through our bodies. If we change any of that energy anywhere in our bodies then it affects some other part of our bodies. If our bodies are affected, then it may affect the energy that is to be passed on to the next generation.

"Another example would be a person who kills hundreds of thousands of people. Many families are thus affected and what would have normally developed cannot take place. The world is now different.

"This interrelationship exists throughout everything we come in contact with, including our own energy and the impact of the imbalance of Yin and Yang as it affects the various meridians and organs.

"Now Pei Ke. Do you have any more questions?"

"No, Master. I think I understand. Actually, I think that what you've said should be common knowledge to everyone from an intuitive point of view. Using your example of the apple, everyone knows that different soils produce different qualities of apples. It's just the way that you explain it that makes a difference."

"Pei Ke, let's take the example of the apple. The Qi of the water and the Qi of the earth and other related examples of Qi, effect the growth of the apple, which gives the apple its own unique Qi, but again, it is all the same Qi. When we eat the apple, we take in the Qi of the apple. Thus, the Qi of one apple has its own characteristics based on the development of the apple through soil, water, sunlight, etc. What would you suspect could happen if the soil of one area was not as good as the soil from another area?"

Pei Ke thought for a moment.

"Master, there would be a difference between the two apples."

"Yes, you are correct. Now, do you remember what the difference would be?"

"Actually, one apple would be more nutritious than the other."

"What does that mean?" asked Liu.

"It means that we would feel better with the good apple than the one that isn't so good."

"But they are both apples," said Liu.

"Yes," said Pei Ke. "But if I understand you correctly, the water and soil affects the later development of the apple."

"Correct. Now think of the things we eat. Each has its own Qi. There is the Qi of the apple and the Qi of grains and the Qi of pork. We could go on and on about the different aspect of Qi for each food we eat. Not only is there the Qi of the things we eat, but there is the Qi of the things we do not eat but which surround us. This extends to both living things and things that we consider not living. Thus, a tree has Qi and a rock has Qi. The interesting thing is the Qi that we humans have, or that Qi which is in non-human things, can influence both human and non-human things. In martial arts, a swordsman finds a sword which is balanced in length, width, and weight. The more he practices with that particular sword, the more the sword becomes part of him. In ancient texts, it is explained that the sword becomes part of the swordsman and is just an extension of the swordsman's arm. You can interpret this as the Qi of the swordsman extending through the sword. Thus, there is the blending of the Qi of the sword, which is metal, and the Qi of the human.

"Now let's take the Qi of humans. Again, it is the same Qi that we have with the apple, but manifested differently. The ancients discovered that salt affects the kidney and bladder. Sugar affects the spleen and stomach. Sour things affect the liver and gall bladder. The lung and large intestine are associated with a rancid taste. Do you remember me telling you this?"

"Yes, Master. But at the time, it was simply factual information without an any context. Now I'm beginning to see the connection between various aspects of energy. I just don't know what all the connections are and how they ultimately influence one another in the grand scheme of our lives."

That night Pei Ke went to sleep with an enhanced understanding of Traditional Chinese Medicine. Liu went to sleep thinking about what had transpired that day. He wondered when the next altercation would be coming and how Pei Ke would respond to it. He was getting tired of this continual battle with Chen Chang and he determined to put an end to it for the safety of himself, Hua Yee, and Pei Ke.

CHAPTER 6

Pei Ke woke before Liu, which was quite unusual. Looking out the window, he saw the first rays of the morning sun coming over the distant horizon. It was the dawn of a new day, the second day on the road back to Liu's ancestral home.

The snow that had fallen during the night had stopped and Pei Ke saw an extensive peacefulness lying over the farmer's fields. At least a half-inch of powdery snow lay on the ground. The snow on the tree branches and rooftops added to the scenic peacefulness. Pei Ke wondered if it was possible for him to just blend into the immediate surroundings and be a part of what nature had to offer.

Scanning the dimly lit farmyard, he looked for the presence of visitors. No new hoof prints or footprints disturbed the pristine snow. It would be a nice sunny day and most of the snow would be gone by mid-afternoon. It would be a good day to travel. He knew it was going to be cold, but he looked forward to being out with nature. He understood why Liu eschewed the fine things in life for the peacefulness of nature. One day, maybe he would be like Liu and able to enjoy the serenity of nature with his master's clarity.

"Pei Ke, you are up early."

"Yes, Master," said Pei Ke as he turned to greet his teacher.

"It snowed again last night, but the weather should be fine today for traveling. There's not a cloud in the sky and there's not that much snow. We should make good time. I think the snow will melt as we travel and so the ground will be a little wet, but it shouldn't keep us from making good time."

Liu walked over to the window and looked out. Pei Ke knew Liu was doing the same thing he had done only moments before. He was not only checking the ground for the telltale sign of visitors, but he was checking the depth of the snow. He had to think about the horses.

Looking at the snow, Liu's thoughts shifted to his attackers. They needed to be cautious on the road back to his ancestral home. Those who had originally attacked and killed his family knew that they were traveling along this road and so they could be lying in wait anywhere. He thought the attack would come sooner rather than later. The farther they were away from his ancestral home, the safer the bandits were from prying eyes and the more likely they would attack.

Even though they needed to travel fast to get back as soon as possible to Liu's ancestral home, Pei Ke knew that, once there, they would soon come in contact, with those who had killed Liu's family. Pei Ke did not look forward to this altercation. He knew Liu would do everything and anything to preserve the life of those he loved.

"Master, we are going to be leaving shortly," Pei Ke said, still looking out the window. He thought he saw motion in the trees and wondered if it was men on horseback, but Liu seemed unconcerned so he pushed on. "But before it gets light outside and we have to leave, may I ask you another question about Traditional Chinese Medicine?"

"Yes, what is the question?"

"Why do patients have blisters?"

"Why do you ask?" said Liu.

"While I was at the hospital, one of the women in the clinic mentioned that one of her close friends had recently had some ugly looking blisters on her abdomen. The blisters gradually dried up and almost went away, but she was in excruciating pain. When she touched the area, it sent pain shooting through her body. Even without touching the area, she felt pain and numbness. It was almost unbearable when her clothes rubbed against her skin. Apparently, the pain was so severe that she had difficulty sleeping."

"It sounds like she has shingles," said Liu.

"What is shingles and what causes it? It sounded very painful."

"Like everything else we treat in Traditional Chinese Medicine, it is a blockage or an imbalance of energy in the body. Some people have this affliction for a short time and others have it for months and even years. It can be quite debilitating."

"How do you treat it?"

"One way to treat this problem is to insert needles around the area where the patient has the pain. In her case, the acupuncturist would put many needles on both sides of the painful area on her abdomen. "But in my experience there is a better way to treat the problem. I would identify the meridian affected by the pain, or in close proximity to the pain. Once I've established that, I would choose one of the major points on the meridian distal to the problem. I would disperse the energy of the meridian by inserting the needle like this." Liu showed Pei Ke how it should be done.

"The patient will probably need several visits to solve the problem. Does that answer your question?"

"Yes, Master."

When Pei Ke looked out the window again, it was much lighter and he saw snow falling off the branches in the distant trees.

"That's probably the movement I saw," he said to himself.

The farmer and his wife were kind enough to provide a little rice and some vegetables for breakfast. After, they said goodbye to their hosts and set out again. The early morning sun felt good against their backs as the horses took them closer to their destination. Pei Ke immediately felt the discomfort of riding in the saddle. Maybe he was forming blisters of his own.

CHAPTER 7

They rode at a brisk pace for many hours that day. Liu was determined to cover the distance from Beijing to his ancestral home in the minimum amount of time and nothing was going to stand in his way. He had pushed the horses hard the previous day. He assumed that Pei Ke was now strong enough in his legs to make the additional effort. He still thought they could make the return trip in about one-third or at least half the time if they only stopped at night to rest. But he kept in the back of his mind the possibility whether or not the horses could make the journey. There was also the possibility of an attack, which could delay them, though he was confident, when it did come he would be able to handle the situation.

Early in the evening, Liu and Pei Ke found a place to stay. As the evening wore on the wind howled and Pei Ke could hear the branches of the nearby trees swaying back and forth, as they beat a cacophonous tune against each other. For some reason, the rhythm reminded him of the drum sticks used in the Lion Dance contests. In his mind's eye, he could see the drummer and the lion-the various beats of the drummer signaling to the men in the lion costume what they were to do next.

The lodging was with a farmer who took pity on them and agreed to provide some food and shelter. Pei Ke was certain the farmer felt sorry for them because of the impending change in the weather. The wind had been blowing from the north bringing with it snow and dropping temperatures.

"Master, we are here for the night. May we continue my studies? Unless you are preoccupied or are too tired."

"My guess is that you have questions."

"Yes, Master."

"Then what are they?"

"Master, you have explained many things to me over these months. I know I ask too many questions, it's just my way of trying to understand. I know we're in a hurry to get back to your ancestral home, but I hope you don't mind me asking all these questions?"

"Pei Ke, we are in a hurry and I do not want to dally along the way, but we can still talk while we are traveling. I will let you know if I am too tired or it is inappropriate to ask questions for some reason. Now, what is your question?"

"Actually, it is a compound question. It's my understanding that the Qi flows along meridians and that when the Qi of one or more of the meridians becomes blocked, there is either an excess or deficient condition which results in a health issue."

Liu had noticed that over the last few months the quality of Pei Ke's questions had changed. Their complexity was indicative of his knowledge and understanding. Liu smiled to himself.

"Yes, that is partially correct. It would be better to say that the blockage of energy in the meridian has caused a health care issue, or a health care issue has caused a blockage of energy. So what is the question?"

"When you insert a needle into an acupuncture point it can balance, tonify, or disperse the Qi of the meridian. How did the ancient practitioners discover that certain points on the meridian had a specific effect on ones' health?"

"Give me an example," said Liu.

Pei Ke thought for a minute. "In the past we've discussed the acupuncture point Tsu San Li. I know that it's on the Stomach Meridian, and it's located on the outside of the leg just below the knee. From what you've told me before, this point has multiple functions.

"As one of the major acupuncture points on the body, it's used for problems and pain associated with the knee and leg. It can help with a myriad of abdominal and stomach issues. It can help with female problems such as breast problems and pain, and menstrual cramps. It can help with a stiff neck, and problems such as headache and migraine."

"Good, you have remembered," said Liu.

"Master, this point is just one of many points on the Stomach Meridian. How many points are there on the Stomach Meridian?"

"There are forty-five acupuncture points on the Stomach Meridian and this is one of those points. Pei Ke, get to the point. What is your question?"

"Would it be correct to say that the energy of the Stomach Meridian, when unbalanced, may cause a health care issue?"

Liu thought for a minute before answering.

"Yes," said Liu. "That is basically correct, even though it is only part of the answer."

"If Tsu San Li balances the energy in the Stomach Meridian, than I suppose the other forty-four points will also balance the energy in the meridian. Is that correct?"

"Yes, that is correct," said Liu.

"Master, if all acupuncture points can correct an imbalance of energy along any one meridian, why can't any of the forty-five acupuncture points on the Stomach Meridian solve the problem of the imbalance?"

Liu looked at Pei Ke. It was a good question, one that indicated someone thinking about what he was learning, rather than simply trying to memorize information.

"Hopefully, he will become a good doctor one day," Liu thought as he formulated an answer that would be in keeping with the level of knowledge that Pei Ke had accumulated. He did not want to make the answer too complex nor did he want to make the answer too simple.

"You are not the first person to ask about the function of one point along a meridian in relation to other points along the same meridian. I remember thinking about that same question when I first started learning Traditional Chinese Medicine. There are numerous answers, but they might not be consistent; they may even appear to be contradictory.

"First of all, the acupuncture points were not discovered all at the same time. Since the initial discovery, acupuncturists have been adding points to their overall classification until we have the basic number of three hundred sixty-one acupuncture points on the body. These three hundred sixty-one points are along the main meridians. There are other acupuncture points, referred to as Ashi Points, as I believe we've discussed, but they are not on the meridians and therefore not part of any one specific meridian.

"Ancient acupuncturists found the main points through trial and error, based on the feedback received from their patients. Patients experienced the Da Chi feeling of the needle and described the energy going to a certain location on their body. In this way, the pathway was established. Palpating along the pathway in some instances would reveal tender points that later became known acupuncture points. I have alluded to this in the past."

"Yes, Master," said Pei Ke. "I understand what you are telling me."

"The ancient acupuncturists found that certain of the points they discovered had a better therapeutic effect on the patient than other points on the same meridian. They remembered this information and later recorded the information and that is what we now have in many of the ancient texts."

"Yes, Master, this is what I am asking. How did they understand this mechanism in ancient times? In my mind, since each point will balance the energy in the meridian, it shouldn't make any difference which point is used. Why do we need to know all the points? Isn't it enough to know only one so that it balances the meridian?"

"In theory you are correct. All we need to do is to balance the energy along the meridian and the body should return to a balanced state. However, it doesn't always work that way. There are many instances where the acupuncturist does not insert the needle correctly and misses the point, but does make a connection with the meridian. In this instance, it is possible for the needle to have a positive effect on the energy, but it will not be as effective as one going directly into the intended acupuncture point.

"Do you remember when I explained to you that one way to think of the energy is to visualize it flowing through a hollow tube in a twenty-four hour circular cycle with the energy returning to its starting point?"

"Yes, Master."

"Let's expand on that concept and visualize that along the way, in that portion of the twenty-four hour cycle that is relevant to the Stomach Meridian, there are hollow tubes within the main hollow tube. Let's suppose there are forty-five small hollow tubes within the large Stomach Meridian hollow tube.

Each small tube goes from one acupuncture point on the Stomach Meridian to one or more specific areas. No two go to the same area.

"Even though the large tube is the whole meridian, the smaller tubes are part of the meridian. Therefore, one point could have an influence over a certain area of the meridian and in turn affect the health issue pertaining to that part of the meridian. This is not how the ancients described it, but it's a visualization that might help you understand and remember the function of the points.

"There is another answer to your question. Do you remember when you first saw me doing Qi Gong?"

"Yes, Master. I've seen you do it many times. We've done it together more times than I can count and I am always amazed at how you are able to generate so much powerful energy. It's almost like there's an internal power you have that's not muscular. You bring it forth effortlessly and at will. It is amazingly powerful!"

"Good. Then you remember that the energy can be projected outward from the palms of my hands. Do you remember?"

"Yes, Master. I remember when you fixed the commander of the troops that were going to abduct us. Your Qi could travel between you and the commander and you didn't even touch him."

"Well, the energy which flows along each one of the small tubes does influence the energy of each one of the other small tubes, and thus the overall energy of the big tube that is the meridian as we know it. That is one way to think of it. Again, it is not how the ancients thought of it, but it gives you a framework to understand it. Does this make sense to you?"

"Yes, Master."

"There is another explanation that might help you to fully understand the answer to your question. The ancients discovered that there are internal pathways branching out from each of the meridians. The Stomach Meridian has internal pathways branching out from the main meridian to the head, abdomen, and leg. One of the internal pathways of the Stomach Meridian actually goes to the Stomach. This is why the meridian is called Stomach Meridian, because it energizes the stomach organ.

"Another way to visualize the answer to your question is to think of each acupuncture point as having a general quality of balancing the energy in the meridian and the special effect of influencing other parts of the body. Thus, we think of using Tsu San Li for headaches. We use the acupuncture point Feng Long, which is four inches below Tsu San Li for treating mucus and chest congestion. Would both points help? The answer is yes, but the Feng Long point has been found to have more specific therapeutic effects than the other point for the specific problem.

"Does this help you to understand why certain points are chosen over other points even though they are along the same meridian?"

"Yes, Master. It helps and I am going to have to think about it for some time. But I have another question."

"Yes."

"Master, you told me once about the Nei Guan acupuncture point, its usefulness, and how to locate it. In our discussion, I remember you mentioning a point called Wai Guan, which is located on the opposite side of the arm. Can you tell me more about this point?"

"Do you remember what I told you about Nei Guan?"

"Yes, Master. The point is useful for treating heart problems, chest pains, insomnia, nausea, morning sickness, sea sickness, motion sickness, wrist and elbow pain, and calming the mind."

"Good," said Liu. "Do you remember how to locate the point?"

Pei Ke placed fingers of his right hand to the inside of his left wrist to locate the Nei Guan acupuncture point. He looked up at Liu for his approval.

Liu looked carefully to make sure that Pei Ke had done it correctly. "Good," said Liu. "Do you remember which point this can be combined with to balance the energy more effectively?"

Pei Ke thought for a moment.

"Master, it can be combined with Gong Sun acupuncture point to treat a wide range of heart problems. In many instances, the combination of the two points Nei Guan and Gong Sun is more effective than using Nei Guan by itself."

"Good," said Liu.

There was a moment of silence. Pei Ke was ready for Liu to continue giving information, but noticed that Liu was deep in thought. He wondered if maybe his master had forgotten that he was going to share more information.

After a couple of minutes, Liu seemed to come out of his momentary lapse of memory.

"Pei Ke, we were discussing the Wai Guan acupuncture point. Is that correct?"

"Yes, Master. You were going to share with some information about that point. Since you taught me about Nei Guan you felt it would be appropriate to also share information about Wai Guan."

"Wai Guan is called the Outer Pass. It is the Connecting Point of the meridian, and the Confluent Point of the Yang Linking Meridian. It is located on the lateral side of the arm opposite Nei Guan. In fact, there are some protocols where you can insert a needle into Wei Guan and connect it to Nei Guan, though this requires you to be quite proficient in your needling technique."

"Master, what is this point used for?"

"It can be used to treat constipation, pain in the arm and wrist, shoulder pain, and any discomfort in the abdominal area. It is one of the Turtle Points. It is used with Zu Lin Qi for the treatment of any problems along the Triple Warmer and Gall Bladder Meridians.

Pei Ke thought about what Liu had told him. He understood the answers to his question, but it didn't seem to be a complete answer. He wondered why his master had paused so long before answering and made a mental note to ask the question again, perhaps in a different way.

"Pei Ke, this is enough for one evening. We both need to get some rest before we continue in the morning."

CHAPTER 8

They had been traveling most of the day. The terrain was quite level and Liu took advantage of it. All day he had urged the horses to move as fast as possible. He actually felt sorry for them. He patted his horse on the neck many times during the day hoping the horse would understand the need to travel so fast. Late in the day as the sun was just about to dip under the horizon, they rounded a corner in the road and Liu saw a familiar sight.

"Pei Ke, do you remember this place?"

"Yes, Master. We spent some time here on our last trip. This is the place where you defeated those bandits who were stealing from and intimidating the villagers. We actually spent a couple of days here and you treated many of the residents. I learned a lot from that experience."

Liu stopped his horse and looked around. Everything seemed normal and he did not sense anything abnormal about the Universal Energy. He nudged the horse forward and Pei Ke followed. They entered the village the same way they had entered it weeks before, but this time it was different. They were not met by armed bandits, nor did they see the villagers being huddled into the center of the village. Instead, they saw a couple of people leisurely walking around the village. When they saw the visitors, however, they stopped and then hurried away. Moments later, villagers appeared from different areas of the village with pitchforks and clubs.

Surprised, Liu and Pei Ke stopped their horses a hundred feet from the villagers, who were now forming a solid blockade. Liu dismounted and Pei Ke followed his lead. Liu handed Pei Ke his reins, then walked slowly towards the group.

One of the men in the group stepped forward, then stopped and turned to those who were behind him.

"It's Liu Bin and Pei Ke," he shouted.

He ran up to Liu and bowed low. There was a cheer from the group and they all ran forward and bowed as well. The commotion drew a response from the other villagers. Doors opened as the group shouted Liu's name to everyone. Pei Ke had never seen such a response like this in his whole life.

"Mr. Yang, how are you?" said Liu.

"Master Liu it is such a pleasure to see you and Pei Ke again. You must stay with us tonight."

"Actually, that is what we would like to do if you don't mind. We have been traveling since early this morning, and we are tired. As you can surely see, our horses are tired as well. They need a rest and some good food and water."

"We will certainly take care of the horses. Have you eaten?"

"We have not eaten since early this morning. If it is not too much of a bother, we both would be indebted to you."

"We are the ones who are indebted to you," said Yang. "If it was not for you showing up like you did, we would still be under the yoke of those bandits. As it is now, we are free of their influence. There isn't a day that goes by that someone in the village wonders if you are ever going to return. It is such a joyous occasion to have you back."

"It is a pleasure to be back. We enjoyed our stay with you before. Your hospitality was as appreciated then as it is now."

"How long will you be staying?" asked Yang. "Please say that you have decided to make this your permanent home."

"Unfortunately, we cannot stay long. We must leave early in the morning. I have personal business and must attend to it as soon as possible."

Liu turned to look at Pei Ke. One of the villagers was taking the horses and walking them away.

"Master, do not worry," said Yang. "Your horses will be taken care of properly. The man taking your horses has many of his own. He knows what to do with them. I am sure he will rub them down and make sure that they get enough water and grain. Everyone in the village appreciates what you have done for us. You will be able to get them as early in the morning as you wish. Now come and let's get you something to eat and a place to stay."

Walking toward the center of the village, the villagers crowded around them making it almost impossible to walk. They all had so many questions that Liu did not know where to start. Nearing the place where they had stayed weeks before, Liu turned to the group, which had become even larger now that the word had spread that the master had returned.

"We want to thank you for your hospitality. I know we have treated many of you when we were here last time and many of you want to ask questions, but unfortunately, we are both exhausted and just need to rest. We need to be up early and on the road. I know you all understand and we appreciate your consideration."

As he opened the door, Mr. Yang turned to one of the women of the village and requested that she put together a quick meal of rice and vegetables and bring it as soon as possible, along with some of her best tea. The woman bowed and smiled at Liu and Pei Ke. She grabbed hold of her daughter's hand and quickly pushed her way through the crowd heading off to her house.

Pei Ke watched as the mother and her daughter scurried away. He remembered the young girl from before. The young girl turned and smiled at Pei Ke. He smiled back and wondered what would have happened if they had stayed in the village the first time they had come through. He knew that more than one of the young girls in the village would gladly have been willing to be married to him. He quickly put the thought out of his mind.

Yang spoke to a couple of the men and then joined Liu and Pei Ke inside the place where they had previously stayed. Liu looked around. Nothing had changed. He was about to say something when Yang spoke up.

"Master, it is really good to see you again. We have talked about you two ever since you departed. You both did so much good for us that we would never be able to repay you for your time and effort."

"I am glad we could be of some help to you. I see you have organized the villagers to protect yourselves from other bandits."

"Yes, we had a meeting after you left and decided that we'd had enough of others taking our hard-earned efforts. We have banded together. So now, anytime a stranger comes into the village, we all come together immediately and show unity to dissuade anyone from taking advantage of us."

"That was a good idea," said Liu. "Have any other strangers come by this way recently?"

Pei Ke glanced at his master, knowing the real intent of the question, but Liu's face was calm.

"There was a group that came by here a few days ago. They did not stop, though. They just rode along the road outside of the village, but as soon as they appeared, the word went out and all the villagers showed up just as they did when you entered. I think this dissuaded them from entering into the village."

Liu realized that he was at least three to four days behind Chen Chang and his men. He needed to travel faster but the horses would not be able to take the pace.

"How many men were there?"

"Maybe ten or more. They were riding at a slow gallop. It looked like they were in a hurry, but not such a hurry that they were willing to wear out their horses. They came by here in the early afternoon, so maybe we were lucky. If it had been later, maybe they'd have wanted to stay in the village for the night."

"You were indeed lucky," said Liu. "I think I know these men and you want nothing to do with them. They are the same men I thought I saw on the hill when we first came here. They are committed to killing Pei Ke and me."

"Master, why are these men after you?" asked Yang in alarm.

"It is a long story. Just suffice to say that the leader of these men has greed in his heart, and his mind is clouded by past events. As long as I am in this village, you all are in danger. You are safe for now, however, as he is traveling west."

Liu started briefly explaining what had happened when there was a knock on the door. Yang went to the door and cautiously opened it. The woman with her daughter in tow brought in the food. She carried a pot of hot tea and two cups while the young girl brought a tray with dishes of vegetables and rice. As they walked past Pei Ke, the mother smiled at him. The young girl kept her head down. As they walked by, Pei Ke smelled the food. It smelled so good and he was so hungry. He could not remember when he had been so hungry. The young girl put the food on the table and the older woman turned to Pei Ke.

"I hope that you enjoy the food. My daughter made it especially for you two. She is a good cook and has learned all of our family cooking traditions."

Pei Ke had no idea what to say. He just looked at the woman who was smiling at him. He looked at the young girl. He thought she was a little younger than him and she was definitely pretty.

"Thank you very much," Liu said to the woman when the silence became awkward. "The food smells wonderful." He turned to the young girl. "You have done an outstanding job. We both appreciate you taking the time to cook this for us."

There was another knock on the door. As Liu spoke to the woman, Yang answered it and then stepped out. When he came back in, Liu knew something had changed. It was not just the look on the man's face. At that instance, the Universal Energy shifted and he knew evilness was closing in. He had misjudged Chen Chang's intentions.

Yang turned to the mother and daughter.

"Would you be so kind as to excuse us now? I would like to talk with Master Liu."

"Of course," said the older woman. "We would be delighted to prepare some breakfast for you in the morning. Will you be staying with us long?"

"We will be leaving in the morning," said Liu. "You do not have to get up to serve us. We need to leave early. Thank you for taking the time tonight."

Yang diplomatically ushered the two women out the door and then turned to Liu.

"Two men have just ridden past the village. They stopped briefly on the road and some of the men went out to meet them just as we met you earlier today. Apparently, they do not look too friendly. Could they be part of the group that you were talking about?"

"I am not sure, but it is likely that the main body of the group went ahead and these two are just following up behind. Or they could be following us from a distance to see what we are doing. In either case, it would be wise for you to post a few men in the village to be on guard tonight. Did you keep the weapons you took from those bandits?"

"Yes," said Yang, "But we are not soldiers and are not trained in how to use them. We would be no match for a well-trained assailant."

"Bring one of the weapons to me. Give the others to the men on guard. Do you have any men you can trust to scout out these strangers' camp? I suspect they have camped on the hill overlooking the village, but I need to make sure that there are only two of them."

Yang left while Liu and Pei Ke ate. In spite of the tension, Pei Ke had to admit that whoever had prepared the food was indeed a good cook. There was a wide selection of vegetables including snow peas, bamboo, carrots, mushrooms, and bak choi. The woman and her daughter had not scrimped at all and there was plenty for both of them. And the tea was certainly of the highest quality.

Before they retired for the night, Yang returned with the information Liu had requested. Liu thought for a long time before finally turning in for the night. He lay in bed until he heard Pei Ke snoring loudly. Then he rose, put on his clothes and jacket, and quietly slipped out the door into the chilly night air. The moon lit the way as he slowly maneuvered through the village, circumventing the men on guard duty.

CHAPTER 9

Liu adjusted the scabbard making sure the broad sword was securely in place. He held it close to his body so that it did not make any noise as he moved from one building to another. He had told Mr. Yang where to put the guards and so it was easy to work his way around them. According to Yang's scouts, men were making camp on the hill overlooking the village.

Liu made his way to the road carefully and quickly. He was sure of what he was going to find, as the Universal Energy, which he relied on for guiding him through difficult times, was consistently correct. There was evilness on the hill, but if he was wrong, he did not want others to know about it.

There was enough light from the moon to help him navigate his way to the road. Here it was a help, but once he found the two men, it might be a hindrance since they'd be able to see as well as he could, but that was like everything else in life. There are two sides to the coin and you have to know which side of the coin you want to be on at any one time.

Walking up the road, Liu thought about the moment in Sun's office when he realized that Chen Chang was going to kill all that was left of his family. Now here he was, climbing a hill toward two of Chen Chang's followers and the rest of the group days ahead of him. He did not know if these two were simply here for reconnaissance or if they had been told to kill him. In either case, he had to find out. He hoped they were alone.

The walk to the hill was not as easy as he had anticipated. It did not look so steep from the center of the village, but when he actually started to walk up from the road, the incline was steeper than he would have imagined.

Half way up the hill, he rested. Even at this height, he could see the center of the village. In the moonlight, he could see the outline of the buildings. At first, he could not tell which building was which, but after a few minutes, he recognized the north entrance and the house where he and Pei Ke were staying.

He could remember when such a hill would have been easy to climb, but now his endurance was not what it used to be. It was very probable he was going to need all his strength when he got to the top. Of course, he knew this was a function of his age. At least he was still strong in body and mind, and he felt he could spar with the best of them at least for a short period of time. Luckily for him, and perhaps unluckily for Chen Chang's men, most real fights were short.

He checked his broadsword then continued to climb. The climb was not going to get any easier until he was closer to the summit. He knew that once at the top it leveled out onto a broad plane

After one more short rest, he reached the top of the hill. The wind blew from the south. Since he was coming from the north, he hoped this would mask his scent, along with any noise he made. He stopped to look around. There was no sign of the two men or their horses. He assumed they had moved off the hill to a more secluded area. This is what he would have done.

The southern part of the hill was forested, which was an ideal place for a camp, especially in the wind. He started toward the trees, but stopped when he caught the faint smell of burning wood. Because of the direction of the wind, it could not have come from the village. When he approached the edge of the forest, the campfire smell was stronger, and he knew he was heading in the right direction.

About twenty feet into the forest, he saw the soft glow of a dying campfire. Close to the campfire were the horses, but they were tethered facing away from the campfire and from him. He didn't think they'd hear or smell him, but even if they gave a muffled snort, he thought he could get to the two men before they woke up.

He walked carefully making sure he did not step on any branches that would give away his approach. He was no more than ten feet from the campfire when he saw the outline of two blankets close together on his side of the fire.

He stopped suddenly the blankets were down-wind of the campfire. No one would sleep like that, close to the campfire, and in the path of the smoke. Something was wrong.

Suddenly, a stick broke and he turned fast, but not fast enough. The attacker had tripped on a fallen branch and had stumbled, but he already had his sword out and he thrust it toward Liu's side. It not only cut through the outer garments that Liu wore, but it also cut through the flesh of his left arm.

The slicing pain urged Liu to flee, but he stood his ground, embracing the adrenalin that was now rushing through his body. It was not a fatal wound and it would not keep him from being able to defend himself. He was more annoyed that he'd allowed this attacker to get so close. Had it not been for the branch or the man's clumsiness, he could easily have been killed right here on the spot.

It was too late to draw his own broadsword, but the stumbling thrust had put the attacker off balance and Liu took the advantage. He turned to the left and stepped forward to grab the attacker's right hand. He pulled at it to deflect and stabilize the man's blade as he brought his own left hand up as well. With both of his hands on his opponent's wrist, he delivered a swift kick with the heel of his left foot to the opponent's right knee. As his foot made contact, the strength and tension in the man's hand released and he buckled. Liu knew it was an automatic response to a pain stimulus and he did not need much advantage to twist the sword from the man's hand.

Now that he had the sword, he swung it in an arc, slicing through the man's knee, cutting the tendons and causing the man to fall. With one final thrust, the man was dead. He could not see the man's face, but he really did not want to know who it was. This man's fate had been sealed the moment he decided to join the ranks of Chen Chang.

He saw no sign of the second man, but he could hear movement off to his right by the horses. He quickly worked his way around the horses and found the second man.

"Who are you?" asked Liu.

"There are more of us, and you'll never make it back home. There's a reward for your death. Even though you were lucky enough to kill my friend, you won't be so lucky with me."

"I have no quarrel with you," Liu said. "Take your dead friend and go. You will never get any money from Chen Chang. He has given you false hopes of a fortune he does not have and will never have. Tell him that if he hurts anyone of my family he will pay the ultimate price for it."

The man spat.

"You don't stand a chance, old man. Chen is probably already at your village laying claim to whatever he can claim. I'd guess your family's already dead."

"You are being swayed by empty promises of money and fortune. How do you know these even exist? Chen doesn't have the money to give you what he has promised. Take your friend and leave."

Liu did not see the man's arm move. The horse saw, however, and moved its head slightly, which was enough for Liu. He dodged to the side, and narrowly avoided the throwing star the man had thrown. In the dark, Liu didn't even see it, but he heard it whizz by his head and stick in the tree behind him. Liu had seen these throwing stars before. They were easily concealed and they were deadly. There were different types, but most had four to six points and covered with a quick acting poison.

Liu yelled and jumped toward the horses. The startled animals reared and the man stepped back with a shout of his own. As soon as he moved, Liu moved even faster. He closed the distance just as the man drew out a knife from his waistband and thrust it at Liu.

Liu saw the thrust and turned his waist to the right to diminish the attack surface. With his right hand, he deflected the thrust to the right, away from his body, and turned into the attack. With his left hand he grabbed the inside part of the man's right hand and guided the knife away from him. He grimaced in pain from the wound on his left arm but he pulled the man's arm until it was straight and used a Chin Na technique on the man's wrist. This dislodged the knife, which fell into Liu's hand.

But the advantage was short-lived. The assailant dropped to the ground and swept Liu off his feet. As he hit the ground, the knife flew out of his hand. He rolled away from the horses and his attacker, then rose quickly to his feet and settled into a Pa Kua Chang ready position.

His assailant was up as well and no sooner was he back on his feet than the attacker was throwing a punch toward his face. Liu blocked the right-handed punch with his right hand and immediately moved to the right to intercept what he anticipated would be a left-hand punch. Sure enough, the attacker punched with his left hand. Liu blocked the punch and was now stepping around behind the attacker.

For a brief moment, the attacker's back was to Liu and Liu took advantage of the situation. He attacked with a flurry of palm strikes and elbow strikes to his opponent's kidney area. The opponent screamed as the pain shot threw his left kidney area.

The opponent swung his body to the left, his left fist aimed it at Liu's head, but from the way his opponent was turning, Liu knew a fist was coming towards his head. He had practiced internal Chinese martial arts for so long that he could listen to his opponent's movements. This saved him from a fatal blow to the temple. He was in the processing of turning and ducking when the glancing blow made contact with the left side of his head. He felt the slight pain to the side of his head as he turned with the contact of the back fist.

Liu continued turning to the right in a full circle to intercept the opponent's left-handed punch. As he finished the circle, his hands were once again in the Pa Kua Chang Dragon Palm ready position, ready to intercept the punch. He deflected the punch downwards and away from him. This left the opponent with his hands down and unguarded. Liu stepped in and pounced like the tiger form of Hsing-Yi Chuan, a move that almost always ended the fight. Very seldom would an opponent survive such an attack, and though death was not always instant, it was always exceedingly painful.

As Liu made contact with his adversary, he brought up his back foot-a characteristic of Hsing-Yi Chuan. He opened his shoulders and rotated his arms and wrists, coordinating the movement of the hands and feet. This was all done in one swift and fluid movement, all parts of his body working in unison. After he made contact, his opponent just stood there for a fraction of a second as he absorbed the energy from the Fa Jing movement. The man then collapsed and that was the end of the fight.

Liu did not even look at his fallen adversary. He knew the man was dead. Instead, he walked to a nearby tree and sat, surveying the scene.

Chen Chang, he realized, was now hiring skilled martial artists. In the past, he had hired untrained men but these two had been very skilled. He would have to draw on all his training if he was to defeat Chen Chang and his men. He sighed as he closed his eyes.

He wondered if he was already too late. Would Chen Chang go to his brother's house in the valley or would he go to Mr. Wu's house? If he went to his brother's house to look for the treasure, it might give him more time to get home to protect Hua Yee. He hoped he could rely on the man's greed.

Resting with his back and head against the tree, he took a few deep breathes to calm his mind and body. Years ago, he would not have been so tired. He was indeed in the twilight of his years. As he reflected on what had just transpired and what was to transpire in the days and weeks ahead, he became even more tired.

He had been traveling the path of learning Traditional Chinese Medicine and Chinese internal martial arts most of his life. His path was the same path that others had followed long before he was born. These *ancient travels* had provided him with untold amounts of *ancient knowledge*. He had learned things that few others had known. Yes, others knew about medicine and others had learned martial arts, poetry, calligraphy and paintings; but few had learned and dedicated their lives to the study of all of these arts. From this *ancient knowledge*, he hoped that he had acquired the *ancient wisdom* of others who had gone before him. He realized he had spent too much time learning, and not enough time sharing and teaching others what he had learned for so many years.

Minutes later, Liu pushed his body away from the tree and walked slowly to where the horses were tethered. He did not want to startle them, so he spoke softly, reassuring them, that it was all right and that he meant no harm to them. He patted them and stroked their manes. He looked them each in the eye and smiled. He made sure the reins were tight and well connected to the tree. He looked down at the dead man and then at the horses again. He had hoped the dead man had not been cruel to the horses.

He grabbed the arm of the dead man who lay at his feet and dragged him to where the other man lay. He would have preferred to carry the man, but he did not have the strength. He meant no disrespect as he gently placed them side by side. He wondered if they had families. He looked at them side by side. Here were two more needless deaths in the name of greed. He asked himself when it would stop. He knew the answer as he turned and started walking back to the village. One of the horses made a sound and Liu turned to see that the horses were ok.

Liu looked at the cut on his arm. The wound was superficial and the bleeding had stopped.

CHAPTER 10

Liu slowly retraced his steps to the village. He was careful not to disturb the men who had volunteered to keep watch. They were not very good guards, but they did give everyone some peace of mind and that was better than nothing.

Quietly, he opened the door to the house where he and Pei Ke were staying. He stood there for a few moments to get his bearings and for his eyes to become adjusted to the darkened room. After closing the door, he took a few steps into the room and listened. Pei Ke was snoring.

He went to the window and adjusted the sash so a sliver of light shown onto the floor to illuminate the way for him to walk without bumping into anything. He had lost track of time, but suspected the sun would be rising in a couple of hours. He needed sleep. The next day would be long and arduous for both of them. He went to his bed, took off his clothes, and laid down on the soft silk lined bed. He pulled the covers over his body as he placed his head on the tea-filled pillow. He was exhausted. His thoughts were with Hua Yee. He hoped she was safe. He mentally sent a message to her to hold on and to not be afraid. He was coming. He touched his arm where the sword had cut him. If felt warm.

Just before falling asleep, he thought of the two horses, still tethered to the tree. He debated whether or not he should have taken the horses.

They were much better than the two that he had purchased. He quickly put those thoughts out of his mind. He hoped they would be comfortable for the night.

The volunteer guards continued making their rounds through the village, totally oblivious that Liu had come and gone during the night.

CHAPTER 11

Pei Ke awoke from his deep sleep as the sun was rising above the horizon. It's rays shone through cracks in the windowsill. He'd been extremely tired the night before. They had again traveled a long distance and he was still not used to traveling by horse. He had been so tired, he didn't even remember taking his clothes off before going to bed. He stretched and sat up, looking around his little room.

He expected to hear Liu moving around in the outer area, but he heard nothing. He was also surprised that Liu hadn't awakened him. He knew they'd wanted to get an early start. At least that's what he said to Mr. Yang. Pei Ke got out of his comfortable bed and put on his clothes and shoes. Something was unusual and he was a little concerned.

He hurried into the outer room and found it empty. He could hear the villagers going about early morning chores and he opened the window, hoping to see his teacher outside, but only saw the villagers.

He went to Liu's room and softly knocked on the door. There was no reply so he knocked harder. When he did not get an answer he gently pushed the door opened and saw Liu lying on his back with his arms crossed over his chest in a very peaceful position. He walked over to the bed and softly spoke to his teacher.

"Master, are you awake? The sun is up and you said you wanted to get an early start."

There was no reply. Pei Ke looked closely at his teacher. The man's chest rose and fell slowly, suggesting that he was deep in sleep, but Pei Ke had never seen Liu so deep in sleep.

He was usually the first one up. Pei Ke bit his lip in worry. He didn't know what to do.

"Master, are you all right?"

Still, Liu didn't answer. Pei Ke moved closer and put his hand on Liu's shoulder, but as soon as he did, he found himself on the floor and Liu was awake and above him, holding him in a painful arm lock. Liu had positioned himself so Pei Ke's arm was not only locked out, but with his weight pushing down, making it impossible to move.

"Master, it's me. I've come to wake you up."

Liu applied more pressure, but when Pei Ke screamed, he realized where he was and immediately released the locked arm. Pei Ke sat up, panting. He was sure that if Liu had applied even a half an ounce more pressure, his master would have broken his arm.

Liu stood up and looked at his student. Pei Ke's face was a mask of fear and apprehension. Liu stepped back.

"Next time it would be better if you did not surprise me like that. You are lucky I did not break your arm or do something even worse. What time is it?"

"Master," Pei Ke said defensively, "I tried to wake you many times. I thought something was wrong. You never sleep so late, especially when we need to be on the road."

"What time is it?" asked Liu.

"A half hour or so after sunrise. The villagers are all up and going about their daily business, but I've not been outside yet."

As he talked, Pei Ke noticed Liu's disheveled clothes on the chair next to the bed. They seemed to have some dirt on them.

"Master, let me clean up your clothes."

Liu looked at his clothes and the cut on the sleeve. Pei Ke saw it also and was about to ask Liu about what he saw when Liu spoke.

"Pei Ke we need to go soon. My clothes are fine."

"But what happened to your sleeve. It looks cut. Did you get hurt somehow? Master you have been in a fight with someone. What happened? Why didn't to call me?"

Liu didn't answer the question as he put on his clothes and adjusted his shirt. Pei Ke could see the cut on the sleeve and looked at Liu's arm. He could see the slight wound. He looked up at his teacher.

There was a knock on the door and Liu held a finger to his lips. Liu walked over to the door and opened it. When he opened it, Mr. Yang stood in the doorway with a big smile on his face.

"We thought you would be gone by now, but I am glad you're not so we can at least send you off with some hospitality. Last night we fed and groomed your horses, so they're all ready. They should be fresh for your travels whenever you want to go." He paused. "Since you have not left yet, does that mean you've decided to stay for a while? At least stay for a day or so and let the villagers have a chance to talk with you."

"Mr. Yang," said Liu. "Please come in and have a seat. I want to talk to you for a moment."

Yang complied, but no sooner had Pei Ke shut the door than there was another knock. Pei Ke looked at Liu, who gave him a nod and Pei Ke opened the door. There stood the same woman from the night before along with her daughter. Pei Ke realized with embarrassment that he didn't even know their names.

"My daughter has prepared a wonderful breakfast for you two this morning. There are vegetables from our little garden along with some rice and plenty of hot jasmine tea. Please take your time. There is no hurry."

The old woman nudged the girl to put the tray of food on the table. She bowed to Pei Ke and then to Liu, which was the reverse of what was the custom, a fact that was noted by Pei Ke, Liu, and Mr. Yang. She stepped back a few steps from Pei Ke and waited. Pei Ke looked at Liu and Liu gave him a stern look. Pei Ke stood up, bowed slightly, and thanked the girl and her mother for the food, telling them that if it was like the previous night's food, it should be delicious.

"Thank you for bringing the food," said Yang. "If you would, please leave them alone for a few minutes while they eat."

The mother and daughter turned and walked out the door shutting it behind them. They were no more than two feet from the door when Pei Ke could hear the mother telling the daughter something. He could not make it out, but he heard enough to know it had something to do with him.

Liu sat down to eat and motioned for Pei Ke to do the same. Pei Ke did not need any encouragement and readily partook of the meal, which was indeed as good as the meal the previous night.

"Mr. Yang," said Liu. "Pei Ke and I will be finished here in a couple of minutes. I know it is not polite to eat fast and then leave, but it is imperative we be on the road as soon as possible. Unfortunately, we have lost some time already this morning and I want to make it up today.

"After we leave, I want you to go to the hill behind the village. You must take two of your most trusted villagers. Two men that you know will not divulge anything of what they see to the rest of the village. Just inside the tree line, you will find two men and two horses. These are the men who passed by the village last night. They are both dead and I want you to bury them. They have no names so no names or information should be placed on or near their grave. There will be some weapons on the ground and a throwing dart imbedded in one of the trees. Use the horses as you wish, the two men will no longer need them. They are now on their own journey into the afterlife where they won't need horses."

"Master?"

"No questions please. Just do as I ask after we leave. You will need to do it soon after I leave in order to attend to their horses. Maybe one day Pei Ke or I will be back through this area and may need the horses. If anyone asks about the horses, just say you found them on the hill, which is really the truth."

Pei Ke was about to ask a question, but he could tell by the expression on Liu's face that now was not the time. At least he could guess where the cut on his master's arm came from now. He ate his food in silence. There was another knock on the door and Mr. Yang went to the door and opened it. In the doorway was a woman who Liu had treated when he passed through weeks earlier.

"I know I am intruding, but I just needed to once again thank Master Liu for what he did to help me."

Liu rose from the table and went over to the woman.

"How are you feeling?" said Liu.

"I am so much better and have been getting better each day. Thank you for all you have done. The gods have blessed you with a remarkable talent."

She bowed low to Liu, turned and left. Liu returned to his food.

"Master," said Mr. Yang. "Is there anything we can do to convince you to stay? Everyone in the village was impressed with what you did to help them with their ailments. This house is for you and your student. We will provide for all your needs." He smiled slyly at Pei Ke. "I am sure there might be some young lady in the village that would be suitable to marry should your student want to settle down here."

Pei Ke almost choked on his food as he first looked at Mr. Yang and then at Liu.

"Mr. Yang," he said as diplomatically as he could. "I am sure there are many young ladies here and in the surrounding area that would make suitable wives, but Master Liu and I must be on our way."

"Pei Ke, finish your breakfast," Liu said.

Pei Ke took the last bit of food and finished his tea. It was truly very good tea. They both rose and went to their respective rooms to gather up their meager belongings. Mr. Yang walked out the door.

There was not much to gather for either one of them and they were soon ready to travel. As they stepped onto the street, they saw a crowd of people waiting. The villagers bowed as the two men mounted their horses. Yang bowed slightly, nodding slowly. Liu nodded as well, glanced toward the hill, than led Pei Ke away.

CHAPTER 12

Liu sensed that something was yet again being disturbed in the Universal Energy and that, as before, it seemed to have something to do with his return from Beijing. He looked around the village. He did not see anything unusual, and though he knew something was not right, he had to move on as quickly as possible. He was thankful the villagers had seen to the animals for the night so they were refreshed and ready to go.

The residents pleaded with them to stay and become part of the village. Liu briefly explained his circumstance and the villagers understood. Even so, they continued to beg even as he and Pei Ke rode away. With all the goodbyes and answering questions, Liu and Pei Ke departed three hours later than expected. Liu wondered if he could make up the time by pushing the horses even harder than what he had been doing. He decided against it.

Just outside of the village, Pei Ke nudged his horse closer to Liu.

"Master, what happened last night? Your clothes are disheveled and dirty, and you look exhausted. And there is a tear or a cut on your sleeve. And what about those things you told Mr. Yang to do? Does it have to do with the men that came through the outskirts of the village late last night? Master, I want to help you."

"I went up to the hill last night. I knew those men were after us and I did not want to have an altercation in the village. There was a fight between us and they lost. As you heard me tell Mr. Yang, their bodies and horses are up on the hill a little ways inside of the tree line."

"Master, why didn't you wake me? I could have helped you."

"I didn't want anyone else involved with this situation. It is better it was done this way.

"Now, Pei Ke, we are getting a late start and we need to travel far today. Unless you have a pressing question, we need to move along quickly. The horses look rested and hopefully they will be able to get us to our next stop before sunset."

"Master, what type of horses did the men have? Were they better than the ones we have?"

"It wasn't a matter of the quality of the horses; it was a matter of being associated in my mind with the evil these men represented. I want to disassociate myself totally from this evil. Riding their horses I would be reminded continually what they represent."

They trotted at a steady pace for most of the day, one that didn't tire the horses and yet still managed to make up for lost time.

As they rode along, Pei Ke thought about what had transpired at the village. He was sure the reason Liu hadn't brought him along to the hill was that he didn't think he'd be able to handle himself in a fight and would be more of a hindrance than a help. He was resolved that if there was ever an altercation he would not let his master down.

They stopped briefly a few times over the course of the day to give the horses a rest. Each time it was at a stream where the animals could get some water and graze on any available grass.

Allowing time to rest and eat, he estimated he could walk ten miles per day. He thought he could get fifteen to twenty miles per day out of the horses, if he pushed them hard, though doing so would ultimately wear them out. And in the end, everything from terrain, weather, and the age of the horse contributed to how far the horse could go. They would just have to judge as best they could when the horses had had enough each day, or they could be stuck with lame horses and delayed even further.

The attack came unexpectedly. Liu saw the two men riding towards them at a gallop before he heard the clamor of the horse's hoofs. It took him a couple of seconds to grasp the magnitude of what was happening and how the scenario was going to unfold. The sight of two men on horses was intimidating. They had an advantage, but there was also a disadvantage and Liu needed to turn it into his favor.

He hoped the horses given to them, had been trained well enough not to get spooked in close combat. He needed to position himself and Pei Ke so the men, who were riding as if they were right handed, had to swing their broadswords across their bodies rather than on the side. Doing so would make the horse pull in that direction, which would make it easier for Liu to pull the men to the ground.

"Master," Pei Ke said nervously, noticing the men for the first time."

"Yes, I know. Get off your horse."

"What?"

"Pei Ke, you are not an experienced horseman and these men seem to know what they are doing. As you can see, they are each waving broadswords. You know I do not have any weapons. As long as they are mounted, I do not stand a chance against these two men."

"Master, what do we do?"

"Get off your horse."

"But they'll just run us down."

"Pei Ke, if you want to help just do it, and do it now."

Pei Ke immediately jumped off his horse.

"Pei Ke," Liu said as he dismounted. "We need to position the horses head to tail and we need to each hold on to the reins of our own horse and keep the head of our horses next to the flank of the other horse. We will be in the middle between the two horses. This will keep the horses between us and the attackers."

The attackers closed the distance quickly and rode directly up to Liu and Pei Ke and their equine fortress. The emperor's horses had been well trained, however, and did not move. The attackers reared to a stop, brandishing their broadswords.

"Hold tight," said Liu. "Let's see what they are going to do."

One of the men yelled loudly in hopes of scaring the horses into bolting, Liu and Pei Ke held on tight. The horses barely moved.

Frustrated, the two horsemen rode around the horses yelling, screaming, and waving their broadswords. Liu's and Pei Ke's horses stepped nervously, but they still did not bolt. Realizing this, one of the attackers backed up, then charged the space between the horses. Liu was facing the man as he rode at full gallop toward the two horses.

"Pei Ke," shouted Liu. "Turn your horse to the right."

Pei Ke and Liu both turned their horses in unison, blocking the advancing rider with the left flank of Liu's horse. The advancing rider came to an abrupt halt just inches away. Liu pushed on an acupuncture point on the neck of his own horse and the horse reared up. The jolt from Liu's horse was violent enough to cause the attacker's horse to also rear up, throwing the rider to the ground. As the attacker hit the ground, he lost the grip on his broadsword and it tumbled a few feet away. Liu dashed toward it.

"Pei Ke," he shouted. Take care of this man on the ground. Do whatever you need to do."

Pei Ke was startled by this command, but he recovered from his initial fright, and let go of his horse. The attacker was just getting up when Pei Ke closed the distance. Pei Ke tried to punch him in the face, but the man blocked it. There followed a series of punches and blocks by both Pei Ke and the attacker, neither one getting the advantage over the other.

While Pei Ke and the first man fought, Liu grabbed the broadsword off the ground. The second attacker was approaching and Liu deftly jabbed the weapon into the leg of the horse. He stabbed only deep enough to get the horse to rear back, taking care not to do any permanent damage.

The attack did exactly what Liu wanted. The horse reared up and threw the second attacker. As the he hit the ground, he rolled on his side. As he rolled, the edge of his broadsword sliced through his pants and into his leg drawing a little blood. The wound was superficial and did not prevent him from immediately standing and facing Liu. The two men looked at each other.

"Liu you are going to die," the attacker said.

With that forceful statement, he lunged, swinging his broadsword. Liu backed up as the man swung widely in large looping arcs and circles. Liu instantly knew that the man did not know how to use the weapon effectively. The broadsword only had one cutting edge, so the wrist action for a broadsword was different then the wrist action of a straight sword. Actually, Liu thought wryly, the attacker was setting himself up for defeat.

On one of the large arcs, Liu stepped in, ignoring the tip of the man's sword as it grazed past his abdomen. With one low slice of Liu's broadsword, the man was dead.

Pei Ke blocked as many punches as he could before one of them made its mark on his face, knocking him backward a couple of feet. The assailant rushed, throwing more punches. Another flurry of punches and blocks ended with a second blow, this one to the side of Pei Ke's head. Pei Ke stumbled again and the assailant rushed him, throwing punches. This time, Pei Ke kicked him as hard as he could in the groin. As the man doubled over, Pei Ke kicked him in the face and then, with the knife-edge of his right hand he delivered a hard strike to the man's neck. Pei Ke heard it snap as the man fell limp. He was dead.

CHAPTER 13

The first thing Chen Chang did when he arrived at the village was go directly to the Liu estate. He needed to examine the compound one more time in hopes of finding some clue as to the location of the treasure.

Riding over the ridge, leading into the valley, he stopped to take in the beauty of the valley and the surrounding area. He relished in the fact it would soon belong to him. He had told his wife and son about the beauty of the valley; and how nice it would be for all of them to live there. He looked forward to the time when the three of them would be together once again.

With one long sweep of his arm, he showed the men what he thought were the boundaries of the land. He led his men down the steep trail into the valley. He remembered his father, Chen Su, telling him about this valley. It had been given to the Chen family by the reigning warlord many years earlier for service done in the name of the emperor. They even had a document delineating the boundaries of the land, and the awarding of the land for service well done.

Chen Chang unconsciously touched the small scroll inside his tunic. While he was in Beijing, he had visited with Sun Han, the official recorder for the emperor, to validate the scroll. Sun Han had indicated that the scroll did not have the official seal of the emperor; however, unless there were other competing claims, the emperor would seriously consider that the land should belong to the Chen family for past service done in the name of the emperor. Of course, all lands ultimately belonged to the emperor and he could do with them as he pleased.

Slowly the group worked its way down the slope and into the flatness of the valley. They turned their horses west and headed for the compound. Chen Chang knew the compound was not too far and even though the sun was descending, they would be able to get there in just a few minutes.

Riding up to the compound Chen saw the closed gates. This was exactly how they'd found it when he and his father had first attacked the compound. That time, it had been easy to get in because they'd had an accomplice inside who had arranged for the gate to be opened for their entry.

This time, Chen Chang was positive that there was no one inside the compound. He knew that Liu was probably on his way back, but didn't know when he would arrive.

Chen Chang had left some of his men in Beijing with very specific instructions to keep track of Liu. If they had the chance, they were to kill him. If they did, they would get a handsome reward. He had not told them the exact amount, but he'd suggested that it would be more money than they had seen in their entire lives. If they did not get the chance to kill Liu, he wanted them to follow him.

CHAPTER 14

Even though he'd been at the temple for several weeks, Chang Song still struggled emotionally with his parents' death. He didn't understand why they were killed. He knew his parents had been servants of the Liu family. According to what his father had told him, and what he could glean from Liu Bin, his parents, grandparents, and his great grandparents had all been servants working within the Liu family.

In return for their hard work, the Liu family gave them a large comfortable place to live and plenty of food to eat. His parents had never made disparaging remarks about the Liu family. In fact, as far as he could remember, they'd always been complimentary about the family, even though they were servants.

During the attack on the Liu compound, his mother gave him the broken amulet to wear, and she had told him to keep it safe around his neck at all times and not to take it off or give it to anyone except Liu Bin.

Liu Bin saved him from the men who had killed his parents and took him captive. He had not witnessed the whole fight that took place at the assailant's campsite. He saw and heard enough to know that one person had escaped the wrath of Liu Bin.

After his parent's death, Liu Bin took him to the gravesite so he could pay respects to his parents. Liu later arranged for him to stay at the temple under the immediate supervision of the head Abbot.

The head Abbot was initially understanding of his situation, but later that understanding changed to coldness and abusiveness. As the weeks went on, however, Chang Song felt the Abbot wanted something from him, and the amulet seemed to be a strong candidate. The Abbot had mentioned it several times. Chang Song had shown it to him when asked, but he was hesitant to take it off from around his neck. His mother had been very clear. Once, the Abbot insisted on seeing it, so Chang gave it to him to look at. The Abbot hadn't returned it until a couple of days later.

Chang had looked at the amulet many times, trying to figure out what was so interesting about it. Each time he felt it around his neck or he looked at it, he thought of his parents. It made him sad that he would never see them again. He remembered the good times he'd had with them. The Liu family had always given his parents time off so that they could do things with their son away from the Liu compound, and he had always looked forward to these times. He remembered fishing with his father in the cold stream running through the valley.

At the temple, it was difficult to get accustomed to the routine expected of him. There were so many rules for him to follow. At first, he would get them confused. There was always a time and a place to do something and sometimes it became monotonous. One of his many assignments was early morning sweeping duties. He was not accustomed to getting up at five in the morning. The monks showed him how to sweep the walkways. He had to do it exactly as they wanted or they would scold him.

He did not mind paying respect to Buddha since he had been brought up Buddhist, but he was not used to spending time twice a day in prayer. The monks made him sit up straight and chant. When he'd gone to the temple with his mother, he had not been expected to sit for long hours, so here his muscles had been very sore since they were not used to the awkward sitting position he was forced to sit in.

Also, the food at the temple was just enough to sustain him. Since the temple followed the dietary restrictions of Buddhism, there was no meat of any kind served at meals. Meals were composed of white rice, one or more types of vegetables, and tofu. Morning meals were usually composed of vegetable filled buns and a hot soybean drink with a little sugar added for flavoring.

There was a strict policy on protocol and who was served first, and who was to do the serving. Since he was the newest member of the temple, it was his responsibility to respect his elders and to serve them tea at meals. The monks would get their own food, but he had to make sure their teacups were always full.

Once the meals were over, he was responsible for the cleanup, again because he was one of the youngest. The monks expected the older boys to make sure this cleanup happened, so if something was done incorrectly, the monks would discipline the older boys, who would in turn discipline the younger boys.

When he lived with his parents he had a separate bedroom, but at the temple, no one had any privacy. He slept on a hard plank with a little pillow in a dormitory style room with the other boys his age. Most of the boys were orphans, or were brought to the temple at a very young age by their parents.

He knew that Liu Bin had gone with his protégé Pei Ke on some sort of journey, but he did not know where they were going or when they would return. Once he'd asked the Abbot when Liu was going to return and the Abbot told him to mind his own business. Chang Song had decided that if Liu had not returned within the month, then he was going to take it upon himself to leave the temple. He was not sure where he would go, but he knew that temple life was not for him. He needed to do something else.

Many nights Chang Song cried himself to sleep. He missed his parents dearly, but knew there was nothing he could do about it. He was thankful Liu saved him from the men who kidnapped him. He was a little disappointed that one of the men had escaped, but Liu had done everything he could do to take revenge on the group who had killed his parents and Liu's family.

One day, when Chang Song was passing through the main temple area, he noticed the Abbot and another man arguing in front of the statue of Kuan Yin. The man looked vaguely familiar, but Chang Song could not place where and when he'd seen the man. Still, he was surprised that the Abbot was arguing with the man. Even though the Abbot was not very friendly, Chang Song had never really seen him angry.

Chang hid behind one of the pillars not far from where the two men were standing. He couldn't quite hear the conversation, but it looked like the man was threatening the Abbot. Chang saw the Abbot nodding in response to a statement from the man. The Abbot was going to raise his hands, when the man grabbed the front of his robe, and drew him close.

Chang Song debated on whether or not he should help the monk, but decided that since the Abbot had been so unpleasant to him lately, he would let the Abbot deal with the situation.

Chang took one long look at the man to make sure he would remember his face, then turned and walked away. He subconsciously fiddled with the amulet. He walked out of the main temple area and went to the outside garden area where the rest of the boys his age were sitting. As he approached the area, the monk who was in charge asked where he'd been. Chang replied he'd had to relieve himself.

Moments later the Abbot walked out into the garden area. He stopped and watched the boys. He started to walk towards the group, but hesitated for a moment and then walked back into the temple. Chang Song wondered if the Abbot knew that he'd seen what had taken place. He thought about it for a moment and then decided he really did not care what the Abbot thought.

On Liu's return, he was definitely going to ask Liu to let him leave the temple. The temple was not the place where he wanted to be. Since he had no parents he wanted to be with Liu. Maybe he could be one of the servants in the Liu household. He could live where his parents lived and help run and manage the Liu estate. Chang Song smiled to himself. He had made a decision and he was happy with it. He just needed to convince Liu Bin. If he was lucky, Liu Bin would teach him martial arts. He could then help defend the Liu estate.

CHAPTER 15

L iu and Pei Ke traveled in silence, both deep in thought. When they took their first break, for the horses to get some water, Pei Ke spoke first.

"Master, it's strange traveling the same road we took to Beijing. I assume we'll pass through the same villages as before."

"Yes, we will pass through the same villages, but we will not stop in them like we did before. We will only stop to rest and get something to eat. We may even have to forgo some of our daily martial arts practice in order to get back to Uncle Wu's place in time."

"Last time, I noticed so many different people. Of course, I knew before there were many different ethnic Han Chinese, but it never really sank in until I experienced the different dialects and features."

"Throughout China, there are over fifty different ethnic groups, and each has its own dialect, culture, dress, and customs."

"Master, what are some of the more unique ethnic groups of Chinese you have seen?"

Liu looked at his student. Pei Ke kept looking around nervously and he hadn't stopped massaging the side of his hand. Liu sighed, regretting the boy's involvement in Chen Chang's vendetta.

"The men who attacked us," he said.

"What?" Pei Ke's voice quivered a little when he said it.

"Did you notice how different they looked from the people we saw in Beijing?"

Pei Ke laughed nervously.

"Master, everything happened so fast. I wasn't paying attention to their facial characteristics."

Liu nodded.

"That is probably a good thing. If you had noticed, you would have seen that they were not Han Chinese."

"They weren't?"

Liu shook his head

"They were from one of the remote areas of this land, a small ethnic group in northwest China.

"We all see the Han nationality group of China because they make up the majority of the population and are spread over most of China. The dialect that you and I speak is the same dialect spoken by the majority of the Han people. Of course, the Hans do speak other dialects depending on where they live in China.

"From my travels and conversations in Beijing, Shanghai, and other large cities, I have met individuals who have their origins with Bai, Hui, Nu, and Zhuang people. You can tell from their features they are Chinese, but you can also tell they are from a minority group. Sometimes it is the wideness of the forehead or the setting of the eyes or the manner in which they laugh or the way they walk or sit. Of course, most people, regardless of their ethnicity, are decent people, though I'm afraid you've learned from your own experience that there are some who are not decent."

Pei Ke was silent for a moment, he then said, "Like the men we killed."

"You mean the men who attacked us."

"That's what I said."

"No, you did not. Pei Ke, listen to me. We would not have killed them if they had not attacked us, do you understand?"

As Pei Ke nodded slowly, Liu noticed he was still massaging his hand and he wondered if Pei Ke would have ever killed a man if he hadn't taken up with him. After a minute, he spoke again.

"I have found that if you treat people decently, most often they will treat you decently in return. Some of the problems we have as a nation are due to a lack of understanding of the subcultures that exist and the uniqueness of the customs within those subcultures. When we do not understand these things, we are often plagued with fear and conflict.

"If we just took the time to understand others, we would all get along better, and there would not be as many social problems and we would not feel the need to isolate people whom we do not understand.

"Look at the religions of China, for example. The major religions of China are Buddhism and Taoism. Those who follow either one of them have incorporated aspects of the other into their beliefs. But there are ethnic groups in China who are neither Buddhist or Taoist. They are Muslim, for example, and follow Islamic customs.

"Still, though they follow Islamic customs, they read and write Chinese characters just like you and me. There are Buddhists who look down on them, but there are also Muslims who look down on the Buddhists.

"The Hui are a primary example of an ethnic group who are Muslim. Their ancestors came in part from the west when merchants migrated from the Arabian Peninsula over the Silk Road. Some of the traders married into the local population and were absorbed into the culture to the point that they speak the same dialect as you and me. They even use the same Chinese characters.

"As you can guess from their past history of trade, they now are engaged in various forms of commerce. They have merged into the basic population, and though they are a separate ethnic group, they are now a part of what we call our motherland."

As he spoke, he discretely watched Pei Ke. Eventually, the boy stopped worrying about his hand, but Liu knew he would have to keep an eye on his student.

Liu nodded toward the horses and they both walked over to the horses and continued on their journey.

CHAPTER 16

aster, we've been traveling for a long time. Are we going to take a break? I think the horses need a rest."

Pei Ke shifted uncomfortably in his saddle, suggesting the horses were not the only thing that needed a rest.

"I agree," said Liu. "We all need a break and we have covered many miles since we left this morning. We will stop at the next stream, where we can rest for an hour or so. Do you remember the farmer who did Qi Gong? You helped correct his posture."

"Yes, I remember. Is that where we will be staying this evening?"

"Yes, if he will have us."

Liu and Pei Ke stopped at the next stream and the horses gladly drank the cool water. Liu and Pei Ke drank as well, and filled the leather flasks given to them by the corral keeper.

"It is amazing how good water tastes when you're thirsty. I can just imagine how thirsty the horses are right now." He looked around. "Master, how long are we going to be resting?"

"Maybe an hour. I do not want to stay that long, but we must think of the horses. You and I are strong and do not have to work like they do."

Pei Ke leaned back.

"Master, while we wait will you share with me more information about Tai Chi Chuan, Pa Kua Chang, and Hsing-Yi Chuan?"

He said it eagerly and Liu looked at him carefully.

"What do you want to know?"

"Well, we've been discussing Qi and the Universal Energy. How does this relate to these martial arts?"

Liu nodded.

"Do you remember when I explained that the muscle meridian system had an influence on the meridian system?"

"I remember."

"When you practice Hsing-Yi Chuan, the moves are basically linear in motion. However, in the system that I teach, there is a rotation to those linear movements. An example of this is Pi Chuan. When practicing the movement, you start with your fists by your waist. Both arms move simultaneously. Assuming you are going to step with the right foot, then the right fist leads, and the left fist is positioned near the inside of the right elbow. The fists and right foot start at the same time. As the fists move away from the body, the arms rotate. We have a linear movement directly forward toward the opponent's head with a rotational movement of the arms. In addition, as your right fist moves toward your opponent's head, the knuckle of your index finger projects forward supported by the thumb. This movement creates a strong forward and rotational energy."

He looked at his student, who was clearly trying to visualize the move in his head.

"Pei Ke," he said. "I want you to do the move I just described. First, I want you to do it as you just saw it. Then I want you to vary the location and position of each arm as you do the move."

"Master, we have done this before."

"I know, but I want you to do it again."

Pei Ke stood and rooted himself, then did as Liu had requested. He repeated the action several times. Then, he began to vary the movements, trying different things. He waited for Liu to offer guidance, but his master said nothing, so he kept going.

Sometimes he rotated one arm without rotating the other. Then he'd vary the movement with the index finger and thumb. He went through every variation he could think of, including moving the right arm first and then moving the left arm.

"Master," he said. "There's a distinct difference in the feeling of stability in my arms and legs as I try the various combinations. Some of the combinations have speed, but no strength. Others have strength, but I don't feel any power. There's even a difference in my strength if I use my thumb and index finger."

Liu watched Pei Ke go through the various combinations. He was pleased that Pei Ke had the initiative to do what he did.

"Pei Ke, which combination of movements gives you the best feeling of strength, speed, and energy?"

"Master, it is the combination that you first had me do. All the others lose speed, strength, or power."

"You can tell the difference between speed and power?"

"Yes, Master. I think I can tell the difference."

"Good."

Pei Ke, felt good about what Liu had just shown him. It was one more piece to the puzzle that he needed.

"Pei Ke you must now feel exactly what happens to both the attacker and the person being attacked. You have learned what positions your arms, legs, and body need to be in and how to both rotate your arms and simultaneously move your arms in a linear fashion." He rose. "I am going to punch slowly toward your head and I want you to use Pi Chuan as a defense and an attack. Are you ready?

"Yes, Master," said Pei Ke, taking a deep breath. He remembered doing this before with mixed results.

Liu slowly punched towards Pei Ke. Pei Ke intercepted the attack and followed through with the opposite hand. Liu attacked repeatedly, each time allowing Pei Ke the opportunity to vary the position of his hands and fists. When Liu saw that Pei Ke had found the right combination, he remarked.

"Have you found the right positions for your hands, arms, legs, and body?"

"Yes, Master."

"Good," said Liu. "Now, let us try Pi Chuan under more realistic circumstances. I am going to punch at you numerous times, each time increasing the speed and intensity."

Without waiting for Pei Ke to reply, Liu punched. Pei Ke intercepted it, grinning as he did, but as Liu increased the speed and intensity of each punch, Pei Ke could not neutralize them. Finally, Liu's attack found its mark on Pei Ke's chin. Liu knew this was going to happen and pulled the punch, but it was enough to stun Pei Ke. He stumbled back, but Liu stepped forward and grabbed him. Pei Ke looked startled.

"Pei Ke, as you surely remember, a real fight will move faster than this. You must be ready for whatever happens."

Pei Ke shook his head to clear his mind. For a second, he'd had a flash of the fight that morning, of the attacker hitting him in the face. He realized that that blow hadn't hurt much more than this, and he was sure Liu had pulled his punch. It occurred to him that he never wanted to be punched by Liu.

Liu stepped back.

"Now Pei Ke I am going to do the same thing as before but this time I want you to use the correct combination of forward movement and arm rotation you discovered a few minutes ago."

Again, without warning, he punched. Pei Ke reacted swiftly. He found that it was easier now to neutralize the attack and to follow through with the counter attack. As Liu increased the speed of each attack, Pei Ke countered. Still Liu eventually prevailed and once again, punched Pei Ke in the chin. This time, however, he shook it off and counter attacked. Liu neutralized it and attacked again, but this time Pei Ke was able to stop it. Liu picked up the speed and Pei Ke responded appropriately.

"Stop," Liu said finally. "You have done well. What have you learned?"

"Master, there's such a big difference between the correct way to do Pi Chuan and the incorrect way. When I do it correctly, I'm able to use less effort and have more power. I am a little slower, however. Why is that?"

"You are a little slower because you are not accustomed to the movement. Once you become accustomed to the movement I suspect your speed will be adequate."

"Master, if we are a system of energy and energy can be enhanced as I have done just a few moments ago with Hsing-Yi Chuan, then this must be true for Tai Chi Chuan as well as Pa Kua Chang."

"Yes, you are correct. That is why many teachers have said that the martial arts of Tai Chi Chuan, Hsing-Yi Chuan and Pa Kua Chang are basically the same. The differentiation is in the movements. You now know the feeling of the movement of Pi Chuan in Hsing-Yi Chuan. Just as Pi Chuan has an energy aspect to it, the other four elements of Hsing-Yi Chuan also have an energy aspect to them. My teachers taught me that because of these aspects, the five movements of Hsing-Yi Chuan are adequate to handle almost any martial art situation. It is not mandatory to learn the twelve animal styles of Hsing-Yi Chuan. Yes, it would be helpful, but it would only be an enhancement to what you have already learned.

"You now know one of the applications of Pi Chuan."

"Master," said Pei Ke. "What are the other applications of Pi Chuan."

"Pei Ke from the front put your arms around me like a bear hug."

Pei Ke faced Liu and did as instructed. He put both of his arms around his master, grasping one hand with the other.

"Now, I want you to squeeze hard."

Pei Ke did as Liu had instructed. He did not want to hurt Liu, so he squeezed lightly.

"Harder," said Liu.

"Master, I do not want to hurt you."

"Harder," said Liu.

Pei Ke squeezed harder. Liu encouraged him to squeeze as hard as he could. As he increased the pressure, he felt Liu's rib cage starting to move.

"Pei Ke, harder," Liu said.

Pei Ke gave it one final squeeze and a fraction of a second later he felt an intense pain in his sternum. The pain was so intense, that he released his grip and staggered back grasping his chest. He looked at Liu, who was just standing there.

"Master, that really hurt. Was that Pi Chuan somehow?"

"It is a variation of Pi Chuan, an effective move against that sort of grab. Just as there is a technique to Pi Chuan, there is a technique to the variations of Pi Chuan. Just because one has learned the basics does not mean he has learned all the intricacies of the movement. Once again, I want to reiterate the value of the Five Elements as a whole system of martial arts. If you can learn the Five Elements of Hsing-Yi Chuan and the variations, then you will in essence know the animal forms of Hsing-Yi Chuan, since they are more or less a variation of the Five Elements."

"Master, my chest still hurts. It feels heavy."

"The contact point on the chest is one of the major acupuncture points in Traditional Chinese Medicine. It treats a myriad of different chest and lung problems. It is also an effective martial art point and one of the main areas used in the Tiger Form in Hsing-Yi Chuan. In this case, I only applied a little pressure, as I know it can cause severe injury, and it is quite painful. It is one of those points where *Fa Jing* can be used quite effectively to quickly end an altercation when your opponent has his hands all over you in close combat."

"Master, what are some of the other applications of Pi Chuan? What you have shown me so far is amazingly effective for so little effort. I can understand why you have such an affinity for the Five Elements of this martial art."

"As I have said, each one of the elements in Hsing-Yi Chuan has more than one application. It is good to know basic applications before learning the advanced intricacies of each of the elements."

Liu ignored the rest of Pei Ke's questions. He preferred to stay on the topic of the energy of each of the three martial arts.

"What I want you to do now is the Brush Knee Push movement of Tai Chi Chuan. Watch as I do the movement."

Liu showed Pei Ke how he wanted the movement performed.

"Pei Ke, now I want you to follow as I do the movement."

As Liu did the movement, he went on to explain it.

"As I told to you some time ago, there is more than one style of Tai Chi Chuan. There is Chen style and Yang Style, as well as variations of these. The principles I will show you will help in learning Yang Style.

"First of all, you need to be rooted to the ground but light in your step. You've shown that you understand rooting, so I will not go into that, but remember, the energy originates in the feet and moves up the legs to the waist.

"Secondly, the movements come out of the waist and flow through the arms. Thirdly, just as the waist rotates so do the arms. Fourthly, there is a Yin aspect and a Yang aspect to the surfaces of the body. The inside of the arm is Yin, the outside is Yang. The inside of the leg is Yin, the outside is Yang. lastly, the angles of the body, including the arms and legs, are important.

"Now Pei Ke, I want you to punch me."

Pei Ke didn't hesitate and swiftly punched towards Liu's chest with his right hand. Liu instantly redirected the attack, stepped in, and placed his right hand on Pei Ke's chest. The counter move was so fast that Pei Ke didn't realize what was happening until he felt Liu's hand on his chest. He realized what a tremendous disadvantage he'd have been in had Liu taken the move any farther than he had. Liu actually was always ready for an attack. He had to remember this, and be ready in an instant, for any attack from any direction.

They went through the same process with a movement from Pa Kua Chang that they'd done with Pi Chuan.

"Now that you have experienced one movement from each of the three internal Chinese martial arts, do you see the difference between the three?"

"Yes, Master, I do feel the difference and I feel the difference when the moves are done correctly. There's a big difference. I would be at a loss to be able to adequately explain the difference unless I'd actually gone through the process and felt the difference."

"Pei Ke it would not be possible for anyone to be able to feel the difference without an experienced teacher showing them how the moves are done. In addition, it would not be possible for someone to experience the feeling unless they had actually done these martial arts for a while. Now let us try it with another move from Pa Kua Chang."

They practiced together for an hour or so. As they did, the horses ate grass and drank from the stream. Eventually, Liu stopped.

"The horses are rested," he said. We must be on our way. It should not take too long to get to the farm. Hopefully, the farmer is there and will welcome us."

CHAPTER 17

pproaching the farmhouse, Liu and Pei Ke could see the farmer chopping wood. A dog barked, announcing their arrival. Two other dogs joined in, each gleefully trying to outdo the others. There was no way anyone could approach this farmhouse undetected. Liu did not remember the farmer having dogs when they had been here before. The farmer looked up. Liu waved and the farmer just stared at them for a moment before recognizing them.

As Liu and Pei Ke rode closer, the farmer strolled to the house and stuck his head in the door. Liu and Pei Ke could not hear what he said, but moments later, his wife appeared at the door, and the two of them walked out to greet them.

"Master, you have returned. It is so nice to see you again. I assume that you and your student will be staying with us again?"

"If you have room for us, we would appreciate it very much. I hate to impose on you once again."

"Master, my wife and I talk about your visit all the time. We were wondering just a couple of days ago if you would be returning this way. I see that you've gotten horses. You can hitch them to the tree, and come in and tell us about your trip. I will take care of them later."

Liu and Pei Ke did as he said and followed him into the house. Despite the addition of the dogs, nothing had changed. It was as if time had stood still, but that was the case in many rural areas of China, where one day leads to the next. The only difference is the planting and harvesting of the crops.

"Master, please have a seat. Would either of you like some hot tea? It's a little cold out there, and in the winter time we try and always have hot water available."

"Yes, we would both like to have some tea," said Liu. They both sat down. Pei Ke was happy to sit in a chair rather than a saddle.

The farmer's wife scurried around the small kitchen area. She realized that not only did she need to prepare tea, but there were two extra mouths to feed that evening. Cups were immediately provided, and extra tealeaves were put in the pot to brew.

"I assume you two got to Beijing. Did you ever get to see my teacher?"

"We got to Beijing, but many of the people I once knew are no longer there or they have passed away."

Liu went on to give a highly edited account of their stay in Beijing, leaving out anything pertaining to their current circumstances. The farmer asked many questions about the city, and Liu answered them as well as he could. The farmer seemed to be quite happy with the information Liu gave him.

"Master, how long will you be staying with us?"

The farmer's wife brought the teapot and poured the tea for the three men. Liu thanked her with a slight bow.

"We can only stay for the evening. We can do more Qi Gong in the morning if you like. It is the least I can do for you for being so kind and putting us up at such short notice."

"I would like that very much. I have practiced every day making sure I did the movements just like your student showed them to me. I am very thankful. I can tell the difference already in how I feel. It is amazing the difference between doing Qi Gong movements correctly and incorrectly. Just holding the hands a fraction of an inch too high or too low makes a difference in how the energy flows."

"Yes. Once you understand the structural integrity part of Qi Gong it makes more sense to the practitioner."

"Master, is it possible for me to ask you some questions about Traditional Chinese Medicine?"

The farmer's wife came to the table and sat down with the three men. She poured herself a cup of tea, than interrupted her husband.

"They have just arrived and are tired. You are asking too many questions. Give them a chance to rest."

"It is fine," said Liu. "I am resting here sipping your tea. Go on ask your questions. I will answer as best I can."

"Thank you Master," the man said, bowing. "We have a daughter who lives in the next village. She hurt her knee a week ago and it is still painful. Would acupuncture help with her pain?"

"In general, the answer is yes. However, since she is not here, there is no way that I can tell for sure. Still there are some things I can teach you that may help her."

"Tell us. I wish she was here now to hear this."

"First, let me ask you this question. What is the biggest health-related complaint that you and the surrounding villagers have?" asked Liu.

"Master Liu, it is probably various pains and injuries. We're a farming community and we work with our hands and backs. Since everything we do is labor intensive, we suffer injuries to our necks, shoulders, knees, or backs. "Quite often when injured, it takes many days for everything to heal, which means we cannot really work." He looked at Liu slyly. "Of course, if you lived here, you can take care of us. We would take care of all your needs, provide you with a place to live, and whatever food you would require. Would you consider living with us? I can tell the surrounding farmers and they could come here to be treated."

"It is very kind of you to make this offer, but I must be on my way in the morning. Pei Ke and I have a lot of traveling to do, and it is imperative that we cover as many miles as possible.

"Since you have been so kind to us, however, I would like to show you how you can help take care not only of your daughter's knee, but of some of your injuries and pain problems as well. Needles would be more effective, but if you do not have any needles then you can use the acupuncture points by applying pressure on the point instead of needling it.

"In nature, there is a duality of forces. There is the Yin aspect of everything in nature and there is the Yang aspect of everything in nature. We all have been brought up understanding this Yin and Yang. This complimentary opposite concept can also be used in the treatment of injuries and pain problems. The ancient acupuncture books indicate that if we have a problem on the right side, we need to treat the left side. For our purposes, we are not going to use needles, but rather we are going to use our fingers and apply pressure to the acupuncture points.

"For example, if I have a pain on the outside of my right elbow, then I need to look for the corresponding sore point on the outside of my left elbow. If I have an injury to the inside of my right ankle, then I need to feel for the corresponding sore point on the inside of my left ankle. You can use this relationship throughout the body.

"This left-right relationship, which is Yin and Yang, can be expanded further to up and down, inside and outside, front and back, and diagonal. For example, if there is a headache on the top of the head, one of the famous acupuncture points is on the ball of the foot. This is an example of up and down.

"If there is a pain area on the upper right side of the chest look for a sore point on the corresponding area of the back. You could also look for a sore point on the opposite side of the chest. You could also look for a sore point on the lower part of the abdomen on either side. Or, you could look for a sore point on the lower back on either side.

"Do you have any pain right now?" asked Liu.

"I have some pain in my left shoulder," said the farmer. "I hurt it chopping wood last week."

"Show me?" asked Liu.

The man felt around on his left shoulder for a few moments, then pointed to a spot on his shoulder.

"Shoulder pain is a very common occurrence," Liu said. "We use our shoulders continuously in our daily activities, especially if we have strenuous or continuous labor intensive work. It is one of the most common conditions an acupuncturist sees during the course of daily practice."

Liu looked at Pei Ke to see if he was following the discussion.

"Based on what I told you before, where do you think we should feel for a sore point?" asked Liu.

Liu listened as the farmer gave his ideas of where the sore point might be located. He thought the sore point would be in the opposite shoulder.

"Let's see if there are any sore points," said Liu.

Liu pressed on the point indicated by the farmer that was sore. The farmer flinched as Liu pressed on the point.

"I want you to raise your arm above your head."

The farmer did as instructed, and Liu could see from his face that he was in pain as he raised his arm.

"Put your arm down," said Liu. "I am now going to press on a number of potential sore points on your body."

Pei Ke and the farmer's wife watched as Liu pressed on a number of points, which could possibly be sore. When he found one the farmer flinched.

"Master, of all the places you've pressed, the last one is the worst. This must be the point that controls my pain, but it is located in a different location than I anticipated."

"This is the most active point for your particular problem. If we had many people here with the same pain problem, likely they would each have a different reactive pain point."

Liu massaged the reactive sore point for a few seconds. The farmer flinched. Liu stopped manipulating the point.

"Raise your arm now," said Liu.

The farmer did as instructed and everyone could see that the movement was less restricted and painful.

"Master, my shoulder is much better!" said the farmer. "This is why we need you to stay here and help us. We are not able to pay you much, but there would be a place for you and your student to live. We could make it a permanent place. We might also find a wife for Pei Ke."

"No, no, no. I do not need a wife," said Pei Ke. "A wife would only hinder my studies. I need to be free to go whereever Teacher goes."

The farmer's wife smiled as she looked at Liu's young protégé. Pei Ke smiled back at her, but did not say a word. That night Pei Ke and Liu shared a meal with the farmer and his wife. After the meal, Liu answered more questions about Traditional Chinese Medicine and Qi Gong.

The next morning Pei Ke and the farmer practiced Qi Gong. Liu watched as Pei Ke once again showed the farmer some of the intricacies of both the static and moving postures of Liu's Qi Gong.

After breakfast, Liu and Pei Ke mounted their horses. Pei Ke settled into the saddle. He was ready for another day's journey.

The farmer patted Liu's horse and thanked Liu for his guidance.

"I think I've learned in just one lesson more from you than I would ever have received if I'd have gone to Beijing to study."

Liu smiled and bid the couple farewell, and rode toward home again.

CHAPTER 18

Master, we've been traveling most of the day. Are we going to take a rest? Maybe the horses need a rest just as much as we do."

"Yes, we will rest when we reach the next village."

"How far is that?"

"It is about two to three hours from here. Actually, we will stop for the evening and visit with some of the villagers. Remember, we stayed in this village on our way to Beijing."

Pei Ke thought for a few seconds and then remembered what had taken place in the village when they originally passed through. He realized that a lot had happened in a very short period of time. Liu was right when he said there were certain times or events in one's life, which would define what would happen for the rest of your life. Pei Ke knew he was definitely on one of those paths. If he hadn't met Liu that fateful day on the mountain, he would be doing what everyone else was doing.

"Master, if we're already to that village, then it's only two or three days until we get to your ancestral village, right?"

"We will try to make it in two days. We can do it if we leave early each morning and travel as fast as possible. It all depends on the horses, and whether or not they can take the grueling pace."

Pei Ke thought about Hua Yee. Based on what they'd heard in Beijing, Chen Chang would either take her captive as a hostage for ransom or try to kill her outright. He guessed he would do the latter and hoped he was wrong.

The sound of pounding hoofs on the ground immediately attracted Liu's attention. It could be nothing, or it could be an attack from some local gang or worse yet, another visit by Chen Chang's men. He could not tell what direction the sounds were coming from. The thundering sound echoed against the pine trees, masking the direction of the galloping horses.

They were in a forest on a dusty and curvy road, headed west. He could see a crossroad up ahead, a short distance from where they were standing. The road behind them curved to the right, making it impossible to see too far that way.

He looked at the forest on both sides of the road. The pine forest was too dense for them to ride their horses into cover. His choices were to stay where they were, ride forward towards the crossroads, or ride back in the direction from which they came. Liu mentioned for Pei Ke to be still and listen carefully. He still could not tell from which direction the sounds were coming.

Pei Ke looked up and down the road, trying to ascertain the direction of the sound. All he could tell was that whoever it was, they were getting closer, and that he and Liu needed to do something soon. He looked at Liu and shrugged his shoulders, trying to seem nonchalant, but his heart was pounding. Again, he saw the face of the man he'd killed.

"Pei Ke, go to the crossroads and continue on to the village. I will turn left and lead them away. If it is whom we fear, they are after me. We have no reason to believe they are after you. I will meet you at the village."

"Master, let me go with you. I can help you. We can both deal with them. You have taught me well, and I need to do this with you."

"No." Do as I ask. Let us go and quickly."

They urged their horses forward at a gallop toward the intersection of the two roads, not knowing if they were walking into a fight. Approaching the crossroads, Liu looked back and saw two men on horseback brandishing broadswords. Liu was about to turn left when Pei Ke cried out.

"Master, there are three of them ahead of us." His voice was shaded slightly with panic.

Liu looked ahead. These three were galloping toward them brandishing broadswords. They were further away than the two behind him. It was obvious that the two in the rear would arrive before the other three.

Pei Ke looked desperately at both groups of men. He could feel the fear starting to well up in him. He glanced at Liu and tried to take comfort in his master's stoic face. Even after all they'd been through together, he still could not believe how calm the man could be in the face of death. Of course, he was Liu Bin. He had nothing to fear.

"Pei Ke, there is a change of plans. We are both going to ride towards the three coming from up the road."

"Master, we do not stand a chance. No, do not go."

Pei Ke was going to say something else, but before he could utter any words, Liu kicked his heels into the horse and it leapt forward. Pei Ke glanced at the two men closing the distance quickly behind them, than he looked at Liu. He couldn't see a way out of this, but he knew if there was one, it lay with Liu. He kicked his heels into the side of his own horse and the horse surged forward at a dead run. This was something Pei Ke had yet experienced before, and for a second, he thought the horse was going to leave him behind. He clutched his reins and for a brief moment, his fear of falling off the horse superseded the fear of those attacking from the rear.

Liu looked back to make sure Pei Ke was following, than urged his horse on toward the three men. The timing would be close, but he thought that even with Pei Ke's hesitation they would be able to get to the three men just in time.

Pei Ke urged his horse forward as he rode into what he thought was going to be a slaughter. He would do whatever he could to help his teacher, even if it meant losing his own life, but that certainty did nothing for the pounding in his chest. He looked back and could see the two men gaining on them. Liu would be up to the three horsemen in a matter of seconds. Pei Ke yelled at the top of his voice.

"Master, I'm coming."

Liu flew toward the three men, and just as he came on them one of the horsemen shifted his horse to one side and Liu rode between them. Pei Ke couldn't believe what he'd just seen. He'd expected a flourish of broadswords and an ensuing fight, but there was nothing.

He cringed and flinched as the three horsemen closed the distance, still expecting to feel steel cut into him in spite of what had happened with Liu, but just as they'd done with his master, they passed him wordlessly, continually brandishing their broadswords. It then dawned on him that these three men were there to help, rather than to attack. They were attacking the two riders who had come from behind.

Pei Ke brought his horse to a halt where Liu had stopped and turned to watch. The two men did not stand a chance against the three.

Liu watched as the fight progressed, broadsword against broadsword. Immediately, he could see that the three men who had interceded for them were not ordinary farmers or rural residents. They used their waists to control their broadswords and they controlled their horses to take advantage of their position. When they parried they never met the attack with the edge of their broadswords. Rather they used the flat surfaces to redirect the attacks. Everything they did, he would have done and he knew that only skilled fighters would be aware of what to do in each turn of the horse. He was pleased with what he saw. He looked at Pei Ke and saw his protégé gawking in disbelief.

The fight was over in less than a minute. The two men who were about to attack Liu and Pei Ke both lay withering on the road. One of the three riders who had saved them dismounted and quickly walked over to where the two bodies lay. Pei Ke watched as he spat on them and then began wickedly hacking off their heads. It didn't take more than two or three cuts to sever the heads from the bodies.

Pei Ke looked at Liu and saw that he was expressionless. Pei Ke couldn't believe what he'd just witnessed. They'd been saved by these three strangers who came out of nowhere in the nick of time.

The man who had killed the two, kicked both heads to the side of the road and then got back on his horse and spoke briefly to his companions. They rode slowly back to where Pei Ke and Liu were waiting, leaving the bodies where'd they fallen. Pei Ke looked again at Liu, suddenly feeling a little nervous. Liu motioned for him to stay put and wait for the men.

The three approached and the leader bowed to Liu and motioned for them to follow. Liu returned the bow and the five headed slowly toward the village. Pei Ke had a thousand questions, but knew he should follow his master's lead, and wait and see what developed. Pei Ke was thankful to be alive. Kuan Yin once again had looked over him and protected him from harm. He would definitely go to the temple when they arrived at Liu's village, and burn incense and pay his respects to the goddess of mercy.

CHAPTER 19

Liu Bin, Pei Ke, and the three men who came to their rescue, rode silently toward the village. As they rode, Pei Ke thought about what had happened. It had been quite fortuitous that these three men came when they had. It could not have been a coincidence, as though they'd known somehow that there was going to be a fight.

They were obviously not farmers. Very few villagers had such martial arts skills as he had just seen. He had a hard time believing that the village harbored three men as good as these. Clearly, these were professional fighters, but where did they come from, and most importantly, where were they being escorted? The biggest question Pei Ke had was how Liu had known they were friendly.

For Liu, the ride to the village was also a time for reflection. He pondered on all the events that had happened over the last few months since he and Pei Ke had left the temple where he'd lived for many years. The loss of his immediate family through the attacks by Chen Chang's father, Chen Su, was the devastating event that started the whole chain of events. He had tried to avenge the useless slaughter by killing the elder Chen, but Chen Chang had escaped and the violence had continued.

As the five horses trotted into the village, a group of men came running up to them. Pei Ke and Liu recognized some of the men from their previous visit. One of these men stepped out from the crowd.

"Master, you are back. We are happy to see you again. You must stay with us this evening. Everyone has been talking about your last visit and wondering if you would ever return with your talented protégé."

As they spoke, the three men continued through the village and stopped at one of the houses at the far end of the main area. They dismounted and tied their horses to the hitching post and went inside.

"Come Master Liu, there are many things we would like to discuss with you. You and Pei Ke can stay at my house. There is an extra room for both of you, and we have some very warm blankets that will keep you comfortable tonight and ward off the chilly air."

Walking towards the house, Pei Ke and Liu recognized some of the villagers. They bowed, and some of them even came up to Liu and Pei Ke and bowed low in respect. Approaching the house, one of the three riders who had intervened for them came out of his house. Seeing Liu and Pei Ke, he started walking towards them.

"Master," said Pei Ke. "That is one of the men who came to our aid. He is the one who is in charge and the one who dispatched both of the riders."

"Yes, I know," said Liu. "We owe him a debt of gratitude for interceding for us at such a timely occasion."

The man walked up to Liu and Pei Ke and bowed slightly to the two of them. Liu immediately knew by the way he walked and the way he carried himself that this man could be a formable opponent.

"Liu Bin, I am Hu Shan. It is a pleasure to meet you. The villagers have spoken very highly of you and your abilities. It is a pleasure to meet a martial arts brother, especially one that is so talented."

He bowed again and Liu returned the gesture. Liu knew that Hu was sizing him up. They each knew the other was capable, but did not know to what extent. Liu had a slight advantage since he'd seen Hu in action and was impressed. When he spoke, he did so with respect.

"We thank you for coming to our aid," said Liu. He bowed again to show his respect and gratitude. "At first I thought you were part of the same group who were going to attack us, but your gesture to get out of the way convinced me you were there to help. I am sorry if we did not help, but I had to make sure I was correct in my assessment of the situation."

"I understand," said Hu.

"Hu, I want you to meet Pei Ke. He is traveling with me."

Pei Ke bowed to Hu, but Hu did not respond. He only smiled a little and continued with his conversation with Liu.

"The villagers have told me about you helping them in their time of need. Your efforts were the catalyst for them to hire me and my two brothers to guard the village for a couple of months to make sure they can live in peace."

"How did you know we were on the road heading to the village?" asked Liu.

"We did not know it was you. The two men on the road were mistaken for some others who'd passed through here a few days ago. They were in a hurry, but from the look of them, they were not the type that belonged here. At the instructions of the elders, we asked them to leave. They wanted to stay the night, but we insisted they continue. Even though we were outnumbered, we got our message across and they left. However, during the night they came into the village, and stole some chickens and tried to attack and rape one of the young women.

"We were out patrolling the area when we saw you two. At first, we thought you were part of that same group, but as we approached you, I realized you were simply travelers." He smiled grimly. "The men behind you, however, matched the description given to us by the woman who was attacked and I realized the band must have been staying in the forest. Then, it became obvious they were going to attack you."

Pei Ke nodded, realizing now why one of the Hu brothers had cut off the attackers heads. Death was the penalty for molesting a woman and he'd wanted to be sure that they would never attack another woman. It was also a message to anyone else what would happen if they attacked the village.

"Thank you, again," said Liu.

CHAPTER 20

Hua Yee was usually a deep sleeper, but the horrific sounds flooding through the house awakened her with a start. She bolted upright. The heavy winter covers fell away, allowing the chilly, early morning air to penetrate through her nightclothes. She shivered and crossed her arms over her chest, hoping to protect herself from the coldness. She shook her head. She was sure she had been awakened by screams from somewhere within the house, and they were close by.

She had retired early to bed that cold blistery winter night and had quickly fallen into a deep, but dream-disturbed sleep. She'd never had trouble falling asleep. As a young girl, her mother often sang to her for a few minutes each evening. She missed hearing those beautiful and soothing words and she counted herself fortunate that she always could fall asleep after just a few minutes. She'd sympathized with those who laid awake for hours each night waiting for sleep to arrive.

In the past, her dreams had always been pleasant. Seldom did she have a nightmare, and when she did have one, her mother had always been there to comfort and reassure her. This was no longer the case and tonight there was no consistency to her dreams. Places, people, and events flooded through her mind, jumbled into a nightmarish mixture of good and evil.

When she woke, she wasn't sure where she was, but after a couple of seconds of cold air, she realized she was still at Uncle Wu's house. Then she remembered the sad and terrible circumstances that had brought her there. Tears clouded her eyes as her emotions swelled. Her grief brought tightness to her chest and she lowered her head and cried once again.

She'd had cried for days at the violent death of her parents. Now she only cried when there were reminders of what had taken place that awful night. The sounds she heard brought back painful thoughts. These images did not come as often now that time had helped ease the pain, but the intensity of what happened was always there.

For her entire life, she had lived with her parents and extended family in a secluded valley north of the nearest village. The setting was idyllic. They wanted for nothing, but this beautiful world was violently shattered by the intrusion that descended upon them. Her parents, along with the other members of her family, were brutally killed weeks earlier by an unknown group of men.

Her Uncle Liu Bin, who lived in the south, came north to avenge their death. With his skills in the internal Chinese martial arts, he had found the attackers and had administered his revenge. One of the attackers had escaped her Uncle's vengeance, but she felt that he posed no further threat, and Liu had agreed with her before he left.

Liu Bin had remained with her for a while making arrangements for the care of the estate. She'd had met his protégé, Pei Ke, and had found him to be quite handsome. Once the estate was secured, her Uncle Liu and Pei Ke had departed to visit Beijing, and she'd come to temporarily live with a longtime family friend who was affectionately and respectively referred to as Uncle Wu. The two families were very close, even though miles separated the two compounds. Uncle Wu was widowed and had no children of his own and always looked favorably on the Liu family and their offspring. Uncle Wu was considered as family.

She did not really remember how long she'd been asleep, nor could she tell if the noise she'd heard had been a part of the dream. She clutched the silk-filled comforter to her bosom. She was certain she heard something in the hallway.

She looked at her bed, and then looked around the bedroom. Nothing had been disturbed. The door was still closed, the windows were shut, and the shutters were still closed. Her clothes were on the chair next to her bed, neatly folded where she'd left them earlier in the evening.

She knew it was the middle of the night and the cool air made her shiver. She adjusted the silk comforter again. She liked the feel of silk and wanted to bury herself into the warmth of the bed. She wanted to go to sleep and have a normal peaceful dream. She wanted her mother and the security that came with motherly love.

With a deep frustrated sigh, she put her head back on the pillow and partially closed her eyes. She liked this particular pillow because it was filled with old tealeaves. The scent was pleasant and the leaves molded to the shape and weight of her head. She remembered Uncle Liu telling her that the scent of tealeaves would help her sleep at night and that was what she wanted now, just to go to sleep.

She thought of Pei Ke, as she had done quite frequently in the past. Uncle Wu had told her they'd be back in a few weeks, but it had been over four weeks now and they still hadn't returned.

As soon as they were back, she would talk with her uncle about getting married. She was close to being of age and she knew deep in her heart that Pei Ke was the one she wanted to be with for the rest of her life. She had seen many of the young men in the area and none of them offered anything like what Pei Ke offered. He was intelligent, handsome, and most important he was loyal to the family. With Pei Ke it would be a good match for everyone. She hoped he felt the same way about her. She doubted her uncle would object to the union, and if he did object, she felt she could win him over.

The last time she'd been with Pei Ke, she'd been certain she'd seen that special look in his eyes that every woman longs for. Even though she hadn't said anything directly to him, she'd implied through words and actions that she was interested in him. She hoped she had not been too familiar. A girl needed to protect her reputation, but she also needed to convey the right message. Since her mother and father were now dead, she needed to chart her own course in life.

She was beginning to descend into the rhythms of sleep again when she heard screams coming from somewhere in the building. Immediately, she was now certain these screams were the noises that had awakened her before. It was not only the yelling of men fighting, but also the horrible screams of people in pain.

This time she knew it was real and not just a dream. The sounds quickly penetrated to the inner reaches of her brain. They were screams of pure terror, just like the screams she'd heard the night when her parents had died. She didn't know what to do. It set off a cascade of emotions. Should she run into the hallway and find Uncle Wu or should she hide somewhere like the last time?

The screaming only intensified as the screams of terror coming from the adults were joined by those of the children. They were coming from all over the compound and they were getting closer. She began to shake and sweat with fear as the sounds closed in around her and she remembered that other night. She wanted to cry out for Uncle Wu, but realized it would be futile. She had been through this before. She needed to escape as she had done previously.

Her first instinct was to get the other children out with her, but the screams told her that they were already dead. She didn't have much time. She needed to do something now. She looked around her bedroom, not knowing quite what she was looking for. There were no places to hide so she had to escape somehow.

Out of the corner of her left eye, she saw lights flickering and shadows emanating from underneath the door. The alternating light and darkness danced wildly across the top of the old wooden floor. Someone or some persons were coming and they were getting very close. She could now hear the heavy footsteps somewhere near her door. Whoever was coming was not worried about the noise they were making. She could feel the adrenalin flowing through her body. It coupled with the mounting fear and apprehension of what was to come if she did not act immediately. She did not want to die. Where were her uncle and Pei Ke?

She jumped out of bed, and ran to the bedroom door and put her ear to the door. Not only did she hear footsteps but she could also hear voices. She couldn't make out what was being said but whoever was coming was not alone, there were others. She thought of her siblings and Uncle Wu. If this attack came from the same group that killed her parents' no one was going to be spared. There was nothing she could do now to help anyone.

She turned and ran to the chair and grabbed her clothes and shoes, and stumbled to the closed window. She fumbled with the cold latch for a couple of seconds before it yielded to her efforts. The cold blistery winter air quickly engulfed her as she climbed out the window and clutching desperately to the bundle of clothes, she jumped into the snowdrift next to the house. As her feet sunk into the soft snow, she realized she'd forgotten her coat. For a brief moment, she stood there ankle deep in snow. Looking back at the window, she could see shadows in her room. If she'd waited any longer, she would have been caught and possibly dead by now. It was too late to go back for her coat.

Her feet became immediately numb from the snow. The icy wind penetrated her thin nightclothes. She could not just stand there and freeze to death. She considered taking the time to dress now, but what if someone looked out the window? Surely, they'd guess that's where she'd gone. What would her mother do in a situation like this? She closed her eyes for a few seconds and prayed to Kuan Yin, the goddess of mercy. She had prayed before when she'd been in doubt, and her prayers had always been answered with the guidance to make the correct decision. After a couple of seconds, she knew what she needed to do, and she knew she needed to do it immediately and without hesitation.

With the faint glow of the quarter moon guiding her, and adrenalin pumping through her body, she ran as fast as she could toward the distant stable. Halfway there, she stumbled and fell face first into the snow. The sting of the frozen ground cut into her right cheek and forehead. Her hand instantly went to her face as she stood up. In the dim light of the night, she saw that she was bleeding. It was not a deep cut, but deep enough that it could easily leave a permanent mark on her face.

She wanted to cry, but knew it would be to no avail. She shivered and knew she did not stand a chance against the frigid air without some warm clothes. She needed to get away from these evil men as fast as possible. They had attacked her family twice now, and on each time, they had killed people she loved dearly. They would not get the chance with her.

Once inside the stable, she sat down on the floor to put on her shoes. She could feel the effects of just a few minutes in the cold. Her toes were numb as she slipped the shoes on. She could not remember being that cold in her whole life. As her eyes adjusted to the diminished light, she looked around for a place to hide. She saw the loft and, with only marginal moonlight, climbed up the narrow ladder. With all her strength, she pulled up the ladder and laid it on the loft floor.

Quickly changing out of her nightclothes, it dawned on her that her footprints would lead directly to the stable. It was only a matter of time before they came looking for her. This was not a safe place to hide. She peered over the ledge of the loft, shaking dreadfully.

She lowered the ladder and cautiously descended. She needed to distance herself from this place as fast as possible, but did not know where to go. If she ran, they would easily track her through the snow. Even if she managed to get far away, she would freeze to death in the cold. If she went back to the house, they would grab her. If she stayed in the stable, they would eventually find her.

As her eyes adjusted to the dim light, she saw the horses. She had helped Uncle Wu feed them. She remembered holding the feed bucket while each horse had taken its turn eating the grains. She looked around the stable.

There were four horses. Two were Uncle Wu's and the other two had come from her parent's compound. Instantly, she knew what she had to do. There was no time to worry about a saddle. She'd have to ride bareback.

She'd ridden many times, even though her mother had said it wasn't lady-like for a girl to be on a horse. Her father had insisted. He had wanted all his children to be able to ride. They were not isolated from the village, but far enough away from it that it was not practical to walk there and if there was an emergency, he wanted his children to be able to ride for help. She'd always been grateful for the opportunity, but never more than now. Still, she'd never ridden bareback before.

Her father's horses looked nervously at her as she slowly walked up to them. Hopefully, they would remember her and not get spooked in the dark. She petted one of them, then the other. Neither one of them seemed to object to her presence, though she could tell they knew something was wrong.

She'd ridden both horses, but there was one she favored. It was brown with a white patch on its forehead and white patches on its legs. It was smaller than the other horse and probably not as fast a runner, but she felt it was more docile and easier for her to control.

She put a bridle on this horse and walked it away from the stall to the ladder. She climbed the first two rungs and steadied herself. Then, with another silent prayer to Kuan Yin, she threw one leg over the horse and mounted it. It moved slightly as she settled down on the horse's back, but it was nothing she couldn't handle. She petted it on the neck and slowly urged the horse forward toward the entrance.

As she rode out of the stable, she saw two men standing at the main door to Uncle Wu's house. They were not Wu's guards and as soon as they saw her, they shouted and ran back inside. She didn't wait to find out what was going to happen next.

As the horse galloped through the snow covered courtyard, snowflakes streaked along her uncovered face. The horse seemed to know the urgency of her departure and its legs quickly covered the distance. The cold wind penetrated deeply and the snowflakes stuck to her clothes. The wind whipped her hair in different directions. It was bitterly cold and she was not dressed for the winter night.

She felt her mother's amulet bouncing loosely against her chest. She remembered her mother's words about keeping it safe and hidden and she thought again about the night her parents died.

Her mother had burst into her bedroom, put the amulet around her neck and had told her to take the other children to the secret hiding place. She hadn't known then and still did not quite know the full importance of the amulet, but she knew it had something to do with the Liu family fortune. She was supposed to keep it always around her neck and to let no one take it from her.

If anything had happened to her parents, she'd been told to either find her uncle Liu Bin, Wu, or go to the temple and talk with the Abbot. She wondered now if she should now go to the temple, or should she go to the secret hiding place where she had hid before when they were attacked. She knew for sure that she needed to get as far away as possible from the current attackers. She urged the horse forward.

She thought again of Pei Ke as she bounced along. He had one of the amulets; she was inexorably connected to Pei Ke through the amulets. Where is he now; and where is Liu Bin? These and other thoughts raced through her mind as the horse distanced them from Uncle Wu's place.

As the horse galloped forward, Hua Yee wondered who the attackers were. She suspected they were part of the same gang who had originally attacked her parent's home. They have come to finish their evil deeds. Why they wanted everyone dead was still a mystery to her. As far as she knew, her parents had never done anything to offend or hurt anyone. They were respected members of the community and had helped many of the surrounding townspeople. Who would want them dead?

Warm tears rolled down her cold check as she rode away from the Wu compound. She felt the tears aggravating her cut cheek. She was angry and a renewed sense of vengeance rose up in her. She vowed revenge on those who had killed her parents.

It was almost a certainty Uncle Wu and her remaining siblings were now dead. She did not know why they wanted to kill her family. There was nothing she could do now until Uncle Liu Bin arrived. She knew he would come, but when? Would he and Pei Ke return in time to protect her?

CHAPTER 21

Far to the east, Liu Bin bolted upright from a sound sleep. He had been moving through a series of peaceful dreams when a deep sense of foreboding swept over him. It sent chills throughout his body. He had experienced this foreboding numerous times in the past, and each time, he knew the Universal Energy had been disturbed by some form of evilness, invariably directed at him. He did not know what the evilness was as he sat up in bed, but from the events and circumstances of the last couple of months, he guessed it had something to do with his family.

They were all in grave danger, especially Hua Yee and the other children. Wu could be in danger as well, since the children were staying with him. The sense of foreboding became worse as he sat in bed and contemplated the situation.

Climbing out of the bed there was a sharp and distinct peak to the unpleasant feeling. He felt an emotional pain that struck every nerve fiber in his brain. He instantly knew that one or all of those he was concerned about were either dead or in immediate danger of dying. Once again, he had not been there to protect those he loved. Tears formed in his eyes. He walked to the window, somehow hoping to see the many miles to his niece. All he saw was the ground and the trees all covered with a fresh dusting of winter snow. It looked so peaceful and was in sharp contrast to what he was experiencing.

The temperature appeared to be below freezing as he peered through the window of the building they were staying in for the night. It would be another two hours before it was light enough for them to travel. He thought about waking Pei Ke, but thought better of it. Pei Ke needed the sleep, and he needed his own privacy to process the premonition he was feeling.

He went to the only chair in their small, tight quarters and sat with a sigh and a heavy heart. He needed to meditate and calm his mind so he could make good decisions.

He placed his feet flat on the floor so the first point on the Kidney Meridian made contact with the floor. He adjusted his back so it was straight. He lifted his head so his spine was straight. He imagined a string attached to the Bai Hui acupuncture point and it helped to lift his head. Actually, the imaginary string helped to open the energy portal so the Yang energy from the universe could enter into his body through the top of his head.

He closed his mouth and touched his tongue to the roof of his mouth. He knew that touching his tongue to that special point on the top of his mouth would complete the flow of energy connecting the Conception Vessel Meridian and the Governing Vessel Meridian. Once the flow was established, he would be able to command the energy in his body to do whatever he wanted it to do. He touched those acupuncture points he knew would open up the flow of energy in his body.

He put his hands over the Chi Hai acupuncture point to enhance the collection and stimulation of Qi. His father had taught him how to do this as part of his early training as a youth. He calmed his mind and visualized a connection between him, the Yin energy of the earth, and the Yang energy of the universe. He started to meditate. As he breathed in through his nose, he brought the Universal Energy into his abdomen.

He then visualized a group of acupuncture points he knew were important for further opening the energy flow within the body. As he visualized the first acupuncture point, he was rewarded with an enhanced feeling of energy flow. He worked from one point to another. Each point he opened further enhanced this flow.

He then visualized the joints in his body. From experience, he consciously made the space between the joints wider. He was further rewarded with an increased flow of energy. He slowly inhaled and exhaled and did this continuously as he went deeper and deeper into a meditative, relaxed state.

He needed to go deeper to accomplish what few had ever accomplished before. He knew he could position his body to align the meridians and the joints so the flow of the Universal Energy could easily enter his body. However, this was only one facet of what needed to be done for him to accomplish what he wanted. He needed to will the energy to do what he wanted it to do.

As he went deeper, he knew that shortly he would feel his body separating from his mind. He knew there was no real separation of the body from the mind, but he knew the connection had been broken and it was a wonderful feeling. It was a surreal experience bordering on pure joy. There were no words to explain the experience. It had to be acquired on an individual basis.

Once in this state of meditation, he could visualize the events as they unfolded and put them in their prospective places. Whenever he was in a situation where he was flooded with conflicting thoughts and emotions, he would meditate as he was doing now. This was his way to bring peacefulness to his mind and body. Many wanted peace of mind and others wanted relaxation of the body, but Liu knew how to accomplish both and they were not mutually exclusive.

Even though he was deep into meditation, he was aware of his surroundings. Many people who did not meditate thought the meditative process meant one was oblivious of one's surroundings.

This was not true of how Liu meditated. He could understand what was said, and what was happening around him. He was just removed from the reality of what was happening. He was now in his own little world. He knew the feeling from having been there countless times before. Each time he could feel the relaxation process take hold in his body. It was an almost addictive process that he thoroughly enjoyed. He felt blessed he could go into this state at any time. He knew others who had tried and would spend their whole life trying to find what Liu now took for granted. He would meditate to renew his spirit and his mortal body.

CHAPTER 22

The two men ran inside looking for Chen Chang. They found him and the others examining the bodies of Wu and the children. The scene was horrific. There was blood splattered on the floor and walls. It was apparent that the last to die was Wu. Two swords lay by his body. It appeared he made a gallant attempt to defend himself, but to no avail. He was literally cut down by the more experienced assailants.

"Did you make sure everyone is dead? Did you find the girl?" asked Chen.

One of the men motioned towards the front door as he spoke. "She managed to get out of the house and went to the stable. She just rode out of here on one of the horses. She must have escaped when she heard the shouts and screaming."

"Which direction did she go?" demanded Chen.

"She went out the front so I guess she went north. We can follow her."

"That will be difficult," said Chen. "We chose this night because there was only a quarter-moon. We will follow the tracks in the early morning. She cannot get too far in this weather. Maybe she will even freeze to death in the cold and save us from killing her."

"What do you want us to do now? The guards are dead," said one of the men. "Do you want us to bury them or leave them where they lay?"

"What about all the others who were here? There was the old man and all the servants and children. Are we sure they are all dead?"

"Everyone is dead except for the girl. I really think we should go after her now before she gets too far away."

"She is young and won't go far," said Chen. "She did not get a good look at any of us so we have nothing to worry about. They can never accuse us since we were never here. I suspect she will either go to the Abbot at the temple or go to her parent's home. In either case, we will follow the trail in the morning. Tonight, I want us to go through this house and take whatever there is of value. There is no reason we should leave anything behind. If we find any weapons, take what you need and leave the rest.

"But make it quick so we can leave. Take the men, and split up into groups of two and search all the rooms. There has to be something hidden somewhere. This old man has to be rich to have these servants and the two guards. If you find anything bring it to me."

"What are we looking for?"

"We are looking for anything of value. He probably has coins or precious stones hidden somewhere. My guess is whatever he has hidden is either behind a wall or underneath the floor. Look for any unusual markings on the floor or walls. Look under the furniture and the beds. Make sure you look in each room and do not miss anything."

"Should we go to the stable and look there? The girl went out that way. Maybe she took something with her and left it out there."

"I don't think the girl has anything of value with her. She did not have time to take anything. She is what we want."

Chen pointed to one of the men. "Go and see what you can find. Be sure and look at her foot prints in the snow to see if she went anywhere else besides the stable."

The men all turned and left. Chen went to the main sitting room of the house. He looked at the walls and the furniture. There were beautiful paintings and furniture indicative of wealth. The old man sure lived in luxury.

It is not fair that some have the wealth and some do not, Chen thought. Both Liu and Wu were wealthy. If he could find some of Wu's money, it would be good. What he really needed was to find the Liu treasure and make sure there were no heirs left to claim the land that was rightfully his.

Chen knew that Liu was on his way back from Beijing. He needed to make sure everything was done before his arrival. Chen knew he had to focus on one and only one thing and that was the killing of Liu Bin and occupation of the lands in the valley.

Once Liu was dead, he could go back to Beijing and present to Sun Han the document indicating he was the true and rightful owner of the land. It was not just for him, but it was also for his wife and only son. They were awaiting word from him. He would be able to do for his son what his father had not been able to do for him. He smiled as he strode through the house while his men tore apart furniture, walls, and flooring.

CHAPTER 23

Hua Yee could feel the pain in her leg gradually going away. When the horse had initially fallen on the icy ground, she'd been pinned underneath it. She could immediately tell that her left leg was broken. In the beginning, there'd been no pain, but that hadn't lasted. Soon, her leg was wracked with unbearable pain, worse pain than she had ever experienced before. The horse struggled to get up, but it's front right leg was also broken. After wiggling out from underneath the horse, the pain got worse. She was sure her movements had further separated the broken pieces.

She lay in the snow for some time, alternating between consciousness and unconsciousness. She was cold, colder than she had ever been. She laughed distantly at the cold she'd felt in the stable after running from the house. Now as the cold started to work on her leg and reduce the pain, she became very tired. She wanted to sleep. She closed her eyes for a brief moment. Just as her eyes closed, however, she felt snowflakes on her face. She realized it had started to snow again and that the snow would cover up all her tracks. Maybe she would be safe from the men who were trying to kill her. She thought of Pei Ke and the amulets they both wore. She knew she had almost made it to the family compound where she would have been safe. The high pass was just a few hundred feet farther along the pathway. If she made it to the summit, she would be able to see into the valley. If she could only get to the valley then there would be safety in her parent's house.

She started to crawl up the remaining incline determined to see the valley she loved so much. The bitter cold descended. Her mind just couldn't function anymore. She held on to the amulet as she fell asleep. This was a sleep she would never wake up from. She never physically made it to the top. Mentally, her spirit carried her to the top for one last look. She visualized herself and Pei Ke living happily in that beautiful place in the valley.

The horse moved its head again as it tried to get up. It too was exhausted from the effort, and like the rider closed its eyes for the last time.

The temperature continued dropping that night and at the higher elevations, even more snow fell. Soon, all tracks became obliterated. A lone wolf howled in the distance. Shortly thereafter, other wolves in the surrounding mountains joined in their sorrowful ritual.

To the east, another wolf howled. It was a deep sad howl, announcing something ominous. Liu sensed the meaning of the deep sorrowful howl and confirmed what he felt before. There was a rift in the Universal Energy, and it was to affect him and Pei Ke and their family and friends. Their lives would change from that moment forward. How they would change would play out in the days and weeks to follow. He knew that once again, evilness had descended and it had touched the periphery of his own being. A deep coldness went through his body as he felt the energy being depleted from his inner soul.

Pei Ke slept fitfully. His dreams were not pleasant. He dreamt of the evilness he and his teacher had encountered since they started on this journey so long ago. He dreamt of the attacks made against them. He thought of the needless killing that had taken place and his own involvement in the attacks against them.

His dreaming shifted to Hua Yee and Mei Li. He had been very fortunate to have met both of them. Either one would make a suitable wife. As he dreamt of Hua Yee, he experienced an uneasy cold feeling. He felt his energy being drained from him in one massive event. He did not know what it was, but he knew it had something to do with their travels back to Liu's ancestral home.

He briefly woke from the dream, feeling cold, as if snow was piled on top of him. He pulled the covers closer to his body to shield himself from the coldness of the room, and put his head back on the pillow. He heard a lone wolf howling somewhere off in the distance. He'd heard wolves howl before, but not like this wolf. For some reason this howl was more mournful than anything he had ever heard before. Tears formed in his eyes and he attributed them to the cold. A sharp pain went through his leg, but slowly he went back to sleep, wondering about Hua Yee, hoping she was safe. He wanted to see her again. He wanted to talk to Liu Bin about her.

CHAPTER 24

hen and his men rose early the following day. He had posted rotating guards for the night. The men who had to stand guard spent most of the night grumbling because they knew no one would venture out in such weather, but Chen did not want to take any chances.

"Where are we going today?" one of his men grumbled. "We've searched this place and haven't found anything of value."

"Leave the bodies where they are," Chen said. "We must find that girl."

"Where do you think she has gone?" said one of the men. "I knew we should have followed her last night."

"If we had tried to follow her last night we would not have gotten far. There was a quarter moon, and it was starting to become overcast to the point it was pitch black out there. We would have been separated from each other and accomplished nothing."

"Well we won't find the trail now," the man said matter-of-factly. "Not in this snow. So where do you want us to start looking for her? Did she go to the village or to someone's home?"

"My guess is she went back to her home. If Liu Bin shows up as I anticipate, he will look for her either here or at their home.

"Since we didn't kill her when my father attacked, there must be some secret hiding place there and I suspect she will return to it. She felt safe there once and probably will feel safe there again. Liu Bin surely knows of the place, so she figures he will come looking for her there. I'm sure the hiding place will be close to the old house."

They found her near the summit where the pass leads into the Liu ancestral valley. She was on the ground. They would have missed the spot except for the outline of the horse under the snow.

"There is something there," said one of the men. He walked over to the snow covered object and brushed away a little of the snow.

"What do you see?" said Chen.

"It's a horse."

"What happened to it?" asked Chen.

"It looks like it fell and broke its leg and couldn't get up. The frigid air at this altitude probably froze it to death."

"Is the girl there?"

"No."

"Look around the area."

As Chen sat on his horse, one of the men walked up the path leading to the summit.

"Here she is. I see the outline in the snow. I think she has a broken leg. It looks like the horse fell and trapped her there. She probably froze to death. The temperature here last night had to be way below freezing."

"Do not disturb the body. Leave it where it lays. This is very fortuitous for us. We do not have to pursue her and the weather has done a better job than what we could have done."

"Chen, she is holding on to something."

"What is it?"

The man bent over the body and slid the amulet out from between her frozen fingers.

"It looks like a charm or piece of metal. It's attached to a string around her neck."

"Cut the string and bring it and the item to me."

When the man brought it to him, Chen looked at the amulet and recognized it as being similar if not identical to the one the servant boy was wearing around his neck. It looked like it was part of a larger amulet.

From the slight curve on one side and its shape, he figured there were four or five more pieces. There must be some significance to the things. That is why the servant's son had wanted to keep his. He'd known there was some greater significance to it.

It was fairly obvious. The amulets when reunited must contain the secret to the Liu treasure, which meant he needed to get the other pieces. Liu himself must have one, but who else has a piece?

This was really his lucky day. Not only was one of the obstacles to the land gone, but now he had a valuable clue in solving the mystery of where the treasure was hidden. Liu would definitely want this amulet and would do almost anything to get his hands on it.

He looked at the amulet closely and saw some part of a Chinese character on one side. To understand the character, he needed to know what the other pieces had written on them. If this piece had a partial character, and the other pieces had partial characters, there could be a message or clue to the fortune.

He needed to get the other amulets. He was sure Liu had one of them and the servant's son had another. That accounted for three of the four or five amulets. He wondered who had the other one or two. He chastised himself for not keeping the servant's son or at least realizing the amulet he wore around his neck had some value. Of course, when he'd first seen it, there'd been no way for him to realize its value. He realized that maybe the only person who knew who had all the pieces was Liu himself.

He tied the two ends of the string together and hung the amulet around his neck. He felt a burden or heaviness as the amulet rested against his chest. He was sure it was the cold and winter wind causing his chest to feel constricted.

To the east, Liu felt something move unexpectedly against his chest. Not only did it sway back and forth, but it seemed to press against him, as though it did not want to be removed. He had never felt this before.

"Pei Ke, do you still have the amulet around your neck?"

Pei Ke felt for the amulet as he looked at Liu.

"Yes it is right here around my neck."

"Let me see it."

Pei Ke pulled the amulet out of his shirt so that Liu could see it. Liu grunted an acknowledgement. Liu knew it was an ominous sign. There was an unsettling in the Universal Energy. Something had happened or was about to happen to one of the wearers of the amulet. He hoped it was not Hua Yee.

Suddenly he felt very sad and depressed. He was almost never depressed as he relied on his meditation to harmonize his life. He closed his eyes and tried to visualize the extent of the rift in the Universal Energy.

A few moments later, he concluded that what he was experiencing, and what the Universal Energy was telling him, was that the rift was personal. It dealt with his family and him personally, and that he was going to be drawn into a life or death situation, which would determine the direction he and Pei Ke would take in the future. All of his strength, both mental and physical, would come into play along with the mental and physical strength of others, particularly Pei Ke.

He hoped he could depend on the boy when the time came, as the feeling he got from the Universal Energy was that they would be united in their battle. The coming battle between what he saw as good and evil would take place over the period of a couple of days and the result would depend on the focus and training of Pei Ke. Liu hoped he was ready.

CHAPTER 25

The two men sat quietly at first, each absorbed in his own thoughts. They were about the same age, but they had entirely different philosophies on life. The taller of the two was brought up in an atmosphere of abuse and hardship, while the other had enjoyed a life of ease and plenty.

The shorter one sipped his tea. As he put the cup down, he looked at the other man.

"This situation has gotten out of control. You promised me you would solve the problem shortly. I assumed you would have taken care of the situation long before now."

"It is more complicated than I expected. Liu spent more time in Beijing than we anticipated. We even had a very famous martial artist challenge him to see if he could help solve the problem. Even the famous martial artist could not subdue Liu. The man is amazingly powerful."

"I can't have any of this reflected on me. I can't be seen talking with you. I can't give you any more information than what I have already given you."

"Liu will be here in the next few days, unless my men have already killed him."

"That is highly unlikely. You have had firsthand experience with him and you lost to him. Even though he is old, he is one of the best martial artist's I have ever seen."

"That won't happen again. I have enough men with me that we will totally overwhelm him, and that useless student of his."

Chapter 26

They rose early as usual so they could get on the road just as the sun made its appearance in the east. Liu estimated they would arrive at his ancestral village by early evening and then at Mr. Wu's just after dark. He was very apprehensive about what he would find. Because of the Universal Energy, he knew he was too late and that Hua Yee and the others were already dead, but he didn't give up hope. He told himself that there was always a possibility that nothing had happened, that it was all in his head.

"Master, if I remember correctly, we should be at the village early tonight. Are we going to stay in the village or go to see Mr. Wu?"

Pei Ke knew the answer already. Liu would want to go to see Hua Yee and Wu as soon as possible, even if it meant traveling late at night.

"We will take the road through the village, but we will not stop. I need to see the Abbot, but it can wait until later. The important thing is to get to Wu's place as soon as possible."

They rode off side by side along the road. They had traveled for an hour when Liu abruptly stopped and looked off into the forest. He sensed there was evilness in close proximity.

"Master, why are we stopping?"

Pei Ke looked into the woods as well, but he saw nothing unusual.

"Master, what are you looking at? I don't see anything there."

"It is not what I am seeing, but what I'm sensing that has me worried. There is evilness in those woods, and it is directed more at you than me."

Liu looked at Pei Ke and then back into the woods. Pei Ke followed his line of sight, but could see nothing and could sense nothing. Pei Ke wondered if he would ever be able to have such ability to sense danger. It had to come from years of martial arts training, or maybe Liu was just born with it. Whatever it was, he wanted to acquire it.

"Master, why is the evilness you sense directed at me? I have done nothing to hurt anyone."

"It is probably by association that this force is directed at you. We will find out soon enough. Since the evilness has chosen to hide from us, we are not going to seek it. Rather we are going to leave it alone and let it play out. We just need to be extra careful about our actions and where we go."

Liu nudged his horse forward and Pei Ke followed, but he kept staring into the forest, looking for something he was never going to see. He felt the amulet around his neck and wondered why Liu had asked to see it. He adjusted the sack on his back. It seemed heavier than usual.

As the horses trudged on, Pei Ke noticed Liu occasionally looking into the forest. Pei Ke also looked but he could never see anything. After a while, he realized he was never going to see anything and he quit looking. Whatever it was, his teacher could sense it and he couldn't, so there was no reason to keep trying, or so he told himself. The next time Liu looked into the forest, Pei Ke forced himself to stare ahead. By the time ten minutes had passed, however, he'd forgotten his resolve and looked every time Liu did.

CHAPTER 27

Master, it's the middle of the afternoon. Will we be able to make it to Mr. Wu's before dark?"

"Yes, if we hurry, we should have no problem getting there before dark. Have you forgotten you travelled these roads before? We will at least spend the night there and visit with Uncle Wu and Hua Yee and the other children."

He spoke confidently, but deep in his heart, he wondered if they were still alive. From what he knew of Chen Chang, the man would do just about anything to get his hands on the land and anything else that belonged to the Liu family. Men who have killed more than one time have lost their fear of getting caught. They realize they can be executed only one time for their misdeeds, and they become more emboldened and fearless as time goes on. Chen Chang had nothing to lose and everything to gain by killing as many members of the Liu family as he could.

A few hours later, they entered the village through the east gate. This was the second time Pei Ke had been through the gate. He wondered if he would ever be going back to Beijing. He liked the big city and everything it had to offer but felt that his destiny was here in this area with his teacher. He hadn't really expressed concern about what was happening, but he now realized that things were coming to a head. This realization sent a shiver through his body. He hoped that Hua Yee was all right. He felt that this was going to be the time that he was going to be tested to his fullest.

As they rode through the village, Liu nodded to some of the residents he knew. They returned his nod, but then scurried off, as if they didn't want to talk to him. This did not go unnoticed by either Liu or Pei Ke. As they rounded a corner in the middle of the village, they met one of the monks from the temple and exchanged greetings.

Almost immediately and without saying more, the monk changed direction and quickly headed in a different direction from the one he'd been taking initially. That would not have been unusual except for the fact the monk also appeared to be totally surprised to see Liu and his student. Liu and Pei Ke looked at each other, but neither mentioned it; they both understood the implications of the monk's actions.

They continued in silence through the village. It was early evening and most of the residents were home. Even so, it was obvious that the villagers they did see knew something they did not. Liu knew this behavior did not bode well for what was to come, but he had no choice, he knew he had to press forward and take things as they happened and be ready for anything.

Shortly after leaving the village, Liu felt the closeness of the penetrating eyes that he'd felt since leaving the temple months earlier. He'd learned to react to the feeling. It always meant something bad was going to happen. They were an hour away on foot to Wu's compound. Traveling by horse, it would be fifteen minutes, if they rode fast.

"Pei Ke we need…"

Liu never had an opportunity to finish the sentence. The arrow tore through the front of his tunic and slightly grazed his right shoulder. The clothing actually deflected the arrow and the arrow only grazed him as it passed completely through his clothing. Three men galloped toward them and one had a bow ready to shoot.

"Pei Ke, follow me!"

Liu bent forward so his body was lying somewhat horizontal to the horse's body and neck. He urged his horse forward toward the attackers at a gallop.

"Master, wait for me," shouted Pei Ke as he followed Liu's example and leaned forward and urged his horse onward. Pei Ke knew he could not let his master down at a time like this. In the past, there had been situations when he froze into inaction at the start of an attack. He could not, and would not, let that happen now. He needed to swallow any fear, and move ahead with determination in order to prove to his teacher he could be counted on during these types of encounters. He resolved to rely on his training and to do his best, regardless of the outcome to him personally.

Briefly, he saw an image of the man he'd killed, but he smothered it in Liu's words: "We would not have killed them if they had not attacked us, do you understand?"

They rode forward as fast as the horses could go. The archer was amazingly slow and inaccurate. His arrows missed their mark by a wide range falling on both sides of the horses, but just before they'd closed the distance, he got lucky and one of the arrows sliced across the top of Pei Ke's leg.

Pei Ke cried out at the sharp pain as the arrow neatly sliced open his skin. The warmth of the blood contrasted weirdly with the cold of the winter air. He put it out of his mind as he urged his horse forward.

The three men on horseback had chosen to have one of the men first attack with bow and arrow because they did not want to physically tangle with Liu. They were well aware of his reputation, especially if Liu was able to get his hands on you. It did not matter to their boss how they killed him. If they could kill him at a distance rather than fighting him in close combat, it was definitely worth a try.

When it became apparent that Liu and Pei Ke were going to close the distance before the archer managed to do any real damage the three quickly closed ranks so that their horses were almost touching each other. The archer took one last shot and again hit Pei Ke. This time, the arrow whipped past his scalp and before he even realized that it had hurt, blood started to flow down his forehead past his eye onto his right cheek.

Liu bellowed and rode right into the middle of the three men and their horses. They parted as Liu jumped from his horse onto the middle rider's horse, knocking the rider to the ground. The man died instantly as the horses trampled him in their frenzy.

Pei Ke was seconds behind. He did not jump from his horse, but rode right into the horse on the right, causing the assailant's horse to rear up and throw the rider to the ground.

Liu turned his horse toward the third rider, but stopped when he realized the man was riding toward Wu's place and that if he followed Pei Ke would be left alone. Liu was no more than fifty feet from Pei Ke when he turned his horse around.

Pei Ke jumped off his horse and was face to face with his adversary when he saw the knife. The man lunged and Pei Ke backed up and raised his hands to head level to get away from the attack. The man lunged again and Pei Ke did the same thing, taking a half step backwards. On the third lunge, Pei Ke quickly stepped to his left decreasing the exposed surface area of his body, and brought his right hand down hard against the attackers forearm, knocking it away from his own body.

Then he stepped ninety degrees with his left foot and grabbed the assailant's arm with both hands. Opening his shoulders, he quickly turned his body to the right, locking out the assailant's arm. With a quick high velocity turn, he instantly snapped the man's arm. The assailant immediately dropped the knife and screamed in pain. Pei Ke was amazed at how little effort he had to put into the movement, and how effective it was, but he made one mistake. He did not continue with his Pa Kua Chang techniques.

When the man dropped the knife and began screaming Pei Ke assumed the fight was over. But, with his good arm, the attacker brought out a second knife and thrust it towards Pei Ke, catching him on the sleeve. It easily parted the cloth and sliced into Pei Ke's arm.

As he approached, Liu saw the anger in Pei Ke's face, but he also saw the calmness and composure needed to win the fight. He wanted desperately to help Pei Ke, but he resisted. The boy was doing fine and needed to taste more victories of his own, even if it meant becoming wounded. An additional victory would solidify in the boy's mind that he should not fear any man.

Continuing with his technique, Pei Ke went into the Pa Kua Chang ready position and started circling his assailant. He could see the broken and twisted arm and wondered how the man could still function with such pain. The mind could do many things when it was under stressful situations. Fear could temporarily mask pain and that is what was happening now with Pei Ke's attacker. The attacker feared for his life, though Pei Ke realized the man was more afraid of Liu, who he saw waiting calmly around the perimeter of the fight. Seeing his master's calm stare filled him with a surge of confidence.

The attacker was swinging his knife back and forth with his left hand. Pei Ke could tell from the way the hand moved, this was not the attacker's dominant hand. He had already broken the dominant arm.

Liu looked around to make sure there were not anymore attackers and then watched the fight between his student and one of Chen's men. He wished he was part of the fight, as he could see numerous opportunities existing in defending against this knife attack.

Pei Ke began walking counter clockwise around his opponent. He picked up speed knowing his opponent would continually make foot adjustments to keep the attack centered. A few seconds later, Pei Ke abruptly reversed direction, catching his opponent in the middle of a foot adjustment. With the knife in his left hand, the assailant would have to come across the front of his own body to make contact with Pei Ke. This was Pei Ke's opening. He stepped in after a few clockwise steps and deflected the knife away. He grabbed the man's arm with both of his hands and applied a twisting Chin Na move to the wrist. The knife immediately fell to the ground.

Holding on to the man's arm, Pei Ke immediately swept the man off his feet. Liu heard the heavy thud of the man hitting the ground. Liu watched as Pei Ke delivered the fatal blow. A gurgling sound came from the man's throat, and blood trickled out from the corner of the man's mouth. Pei Ke looked into the man's eyes and could see the fear. Seconds later the man was dead.

Pei Ke stood up and started kicking the dead man in the ribs. He cursed the dead man as he continued to deliver a series of kicks to different parts of the man's body. Liu ran up and grabbed Pei Ke.

"Pei Ke, he is already dead."

Pei Ke turned to Liu, and Liu could see the wildness in his student's eyes. Liu had seen this look before. It was the look of someone out of control and consumed with anger and rage.

"Pei Ke, settle down. You have defended yourself appropriately. His death was his own destiny."

As Pei Ke's breathing calmed down, the reality of what happened set in.

"Master, you have taught me that all life is precious and we should do nothing to take another life."

"Yes, that is the teachings of Buddhism and Taoism; and, of course, those are my teachings as well. You should value all life. That is why we do not eat meat or harm others. Your life is also precious and no one should do anything to take it from you. You acted as I would have acted in the same situation. You have learned well. However, I caution you about losing control of your emotions, especially the emotions of anger and rage. Know when to stop and when not to stop. This comes from knowing your own abilities."

"Should I have let him live?" asked Pei Ke.

"If he lived, you would probably have to go through the same thing with him again at another time and place. He had greed driving him. Nothing could have been done to change him. The other attacker will go back to Chen and tell him that we are back, but there are now two less men we have to worry about. We are not attacking them; they are attacking us, and for greed only. I do not know when we will see Chen, but when we meet, there will be an altercation to resolve this issue of who owns the land. We need to be victorious."

"Master, what should we do with the two bodies? Should we take them back to the village or should we take them to Mr. Wu's?"

"Nothing. Let the two of them lay where they fell. They do not deserve any respect. We have done nothing to deserve this attack. It is the greed of Chen and his promise of wealth that has led these men to do what they have tried to do."

"Master, what about the horses? Should we take the horses with us?"

"The horses have done nothing to us. They are as innocent as we are and we do not want to be accused of killing two men for their horses. Leave them for the villagers.

"Pei Ke, with these men so close to Mr. Wu's we really need to hurry.

Liu and Pei Ke examined each other's wounds. They had all stopped bleeding and no major damage had been done. Kuan Yin had looked after both of them.

They rode off toward Mr. Wu's. Neither one of them looked back as the two horses stood over the two dead men.

CHAPTER 28

The man sat in his chair sipping green tea. He had been sitting there for a couple of hours, reflecting on the events that had transpired over the last couple of months. What was going to be a simple association with a common goal had turned out to be more than what he wanted. He was being drawn deeper and deeper into a situation he could no longer control. It had gotten so bad that there was no way for him to honorably get out of it.

He needed to make a decision. This was a decision that would forever change him. It could very well violate everything that he stood for and it could easily cost him his life. He wished he had never been talked into the situation.

He thought about praying to Kuan Yin but realized the contradiction.

CHAPTER 29

The sun was just about to dip over the horizon as Liu and Pei Ke galloped up to Wu's compound. The first thing they noticed was the absence of guards to challenge them. Wu had always been cautious about someone sneaking up on him, so Liu immediately knew something was wrong and totally out of place. He feared for the worst as he approached the main gate. It was unlocked and he pushed it open and entered the main compound.

"Master, there's no one here," said Pei Ke. "Where are Mr. Wu and Hua Yee?"

"I do not know," said Liu as they walked into the compound.

"Pei Ke, follow me and pay attention to what you see."

They walked through the front door of the main house to find the interior in pieces. Chairs were overturned, there were holes in the floor, and part of the wall had been pried loose. Cabinets were overturned and their contents strewn over the floor.

Liu walked toward the hallway leading to the bedrooms with Pei Ke close behind. As he entered the hallway, he saw the first signs of blood on the floor. Further down the hallway, not only was there blood on the floor, but also on the walls.

Their first stop was Mr. Wu's bedroom. Whoever had attacked the place would most likely have come here first. There was no blood on the bed, but there was a lot of dried blood on the floor. It looked like Wu had put up a fight in the corner. When he'd been killed, he'd dropped on the spot. There was so much blood that he must have died from loss of blood; there was not any blood anywhere else in the room. This was in contrast to the blood that was in the hallways, which must have been where some of the guards died before Wu met his end. By the look of the dried blood, whatever happened took place a few days ago.

Feeling sad, they hurried next to the bedroom where Hua Yee would have been sleeping, uncertain and afraid of what they might find. The door was slightly ajar and they felt the cold air as soon as they entered the room. The window was open and just as in the sitting room, everything was strewn all over the floor. There was no blood, however, and they took that as a good sign. If this was the room she'd been sleeping in, and Liu thought for sure it was, then she either escaped through the window or had been captured and was being held for some type of ransom. Liu looked carefully around the room, scanning for any clues, but there was nothing out of the ordinary.

They examined the remainder of the house and found more of the same destruction. Those who had attacked the place had either killed everyone or run everyone off. He guessed by the number of blood stained areas that everyone had been killed. Every room, including the servants quarters, had been torn apart by the attackers. It was interesting that there were no bodies. They were looking for something, but Liu was sure they would not have found it.

Liu walked back to the main sitting room, and sat down in a chair, and put his face into his hands and started to cry. He was sure Chen had done this. There was no reasoning behind the senseless killing.

Pei Ke sat down beside his master and was at a loss for words. He did not know what to say. He wondered where Hua Yee was and if she had escaped the massacre. Tears formed in his eyes and he could feel the anger and resentment building up in him over this senseless massacre. He wished he could have been here to prevent the killing.

"Master, there is no one here? They must have put up a tremendous fight, but they were obviously overwhelmed. There are no bodies whatsoever, in any of the rooms. Who would have done such a thing as this?"

With tears running down his cheeks, Liu got up and walked back to the room where Hua Yee would have been sleeping. He carefully looked around the room, examining everything, including the bed and the area where she would have put her clothes. Everything seemed to be in order. He looked out the window, but could see nothing out of the ordinary. He sat on the bed with tears still streaming down his cheeks. Pei Ke sat next to him.

"Master, I am so sorry this has happened. There are no words for me to express my feelings."

Pei Ke started to cry.

"It was Chen, wasn't it?"

"Yes, I am sure of it. It was such a needless and cruel deed on his part. The Universal Energy will be on my side and he will not have his way in this ongoing feud. I will prevail."

"Master, I am very concerned for Hua Yee."

"I know," said Liu. "I know you had a special place in your heart for her. I suspect she had a special place in her heart for you as well."

"Master, what are we going to do?"

"Tonight we are going to stay here. I need to think this situation through and decide what needs to be done. It is obvious someone removed the bodies, but I don't think it was Chen. I suspect the temple has taken care of them. We will ask the Abbot when we see him.

"Now we know why the monk in the village acted so strangely when we saw him and why the few people we saw in the village kind of ignored us. They knew who we were.

"I suspect that Chen is either somewhere nearby or at my ancestral home north of the village. When that last rider rode off after our fight on the road, he headed in this direction, probably to find Chen and report on what took place. If Chen is camped in this area, then he might come and try to attack us tonight. On the other hand, if he did attack this place, then he would be very unlikely to return especially since the villagers already know there has been a massacre at this location. I believe he is at my ancestral home and we will not have to worry about him until tomorrow or the next day."

"Master, should we set a watch tonight?"

"No, he is not going to show up tonight. We can find a place here at Mr. Wu's for the evening. There must be some food in the kitchen. Why don't you go and see what you can find. Maybe there are some vegetables and a little rice you can cook for us."

"Yes, Master."

Pei Ke went off in the direction of the kitchen and Liu went into one of the bedrooms. It was just as torn up as all the other rooms. Chairs and cabinets had been overturned and their contents lay scattered on the floor.

The Wu family and the Liu family had been close friends going back many years. They had helped each other many times and considered each other as family. Each would do anything to help the other and trusted the other to help in time of need. The trust went so far as to know the location of secret hiding places in case there was an emergency.

Liu knew the location of Wu's secret hiding place. It was in this bedroom where he now stood. Even though Chen's men had gone through the place, they had not known what to look for. The key to the secret hiding place was in the bedpost. Liu could not remember which one it was, but one of them would unscrew half way down, exposing a long thin metal key. Liu tested each one of the posts and found the correct one. Looking at the post one would never see it looked slightly different from the other three. It unscrewed about half way down and Liu pulled out a long key from the hollowed out post.

With the key in hand, Liu went over to the corner of the northwest wall. On the floor was a broken statue of Kuan Yin. He looked at the statue and thought about where the Liu family had hidden some of its treasure. At the base of the wall, he found the small hole he was looking for.

The key was long, and it had a flat surface at the end. It did not look like a regular key that would open a door; rather it looked like a thin flat piece of metal with a ninety-degree angle at the end. When inserted just right into the hole it slid into the wall. Liu inserted the key and gently pushed it into the wall. He felt the key come in contact with something and he gently worked the angled end around until he found the lever. He pulled on the key and a small piece of wood at the base of the wall popped open.

Liu removed the key, inserted it back into the hollow bedpost, than screwed the top of the post back onto the base. He put his arm into the hiding place and pulled out several scrolls. He knew the significance of these scrolls. One indicated the hiding place for some of Wu's precious metals.

Another was a deed to the property given to Wu by the emperor. Another was a will, giving the property on Wu's death to the oldest living member of the Liu family. Liu looked carefully into the secret hiding place to make sure nothing else was there. He put the piece of wood back where it belonged and he heard a click indicating that the lever inside the wall had been reset. He then left the room and closed the bedroom door. He gave the scrolls to Pei Ke who put them in the sack.

CHAPTER 30

That night Liu and Pei Ke discussed the events that had taken place since they had first met on that fateful day on the mountain. For Liu it was just a short time ago. For Pei Ke it seemed like ages ago. He had learned so much about Traditional Chinese Medicine and Chinese internal martial arts. If he hadn't met Liu, he would be doing the same dull things he'd been doing before they met.

Pei Ke once more realized there were defining moments in one's life when a decision, event, or series of events altered what would take place for the rest of one's life. He had made such a decision and now could never go back to his old way of life.

He now wondered where he would be going from here. There were decisions and events that were going to unfold in the next few days that would drastically change his life again. It was like the road to Beijing. He could have taken either road, but he took the road to the left that made all the difference. What would it be like if he had taken the other road? He never would know, and it really did not matter. He was now on this road.

As they talked, Pei Ke realized his teacher was opening up to him, including him in some of his most private thoughts and personal feelings. He felt Liu had let down a barrier that had existed between them. There was still a teacher-student relationship, and there always would be, but Liu was formal and more like a guide than a taskmaster.

Pei Ke knew this relationship only came about because of everything they'd experienced together and the trust those experiences had created. Pei Ke worked hard for that trust and he promised himself that he would do nothing to violate it.

"Master, where are we going to sleep? Can we use some of the bedrooms or are we going to sleep in the main sitting room?"

"I am going to sleep in one of the rooms where no one was killed. I do not want to be around the energy of death and you can sleep down the hallway in Hua Yee's room. There is no sign of death in her room. You can sleep in her bed; it will be comfortable for you. I choose to sleep on the wood floor."

"What time will we be getting up in the morning?"

"I do not know. There are many things I need to think about tonight, and it depends on how tired I am in the morning. The last few days have been both physically demanding and emotionally tiring for me. You need to get a good night's rest too. You've had your own set of trials and tomorrow will be more strenuous than you think. Chen is out there somewhere and he may have men ready at different locations to ambush us."

"Master, we should travel south to see Wei Ken De. Maybe he can help us to defeat Chen and his men. With our horses, it wouldn't take us that much time to get to his place. We could spend the night and discuss the situation with him. If he joined us, we'd be in a better position to handle the evilness of Chen. Do you think he would be willing to help us?"

"That is a very good idea. I never thought about it. It would be to our advantage to have another martial artist with us, and he is very good. I am sure he would be willing to help us. Let me give some consideration to what you have suggested."

Pei Ke thought Wei Ken De was just the man to help. He was very direct and from the little Pei Ke had seen of his Hsing-Yi Chuan and Pa Kua Chang, Chen's men would have to be exceptionally good to defeat him.

Despite his grief, worry, and weariness, when he finally went to sleep, he was smiling that he'd suggested something that could truly help his master.

CHAPTER 31

Liu and Pei Ke timed their arrival at the temple to correspond with the end of breakfast. Liu wanted to talk with the Abbot before he became involved in his daily activities. On their arrival, they immediately went to the Abbot's office where they were greeted by his assistant.

"Master Liu, I am so sorry to hear about what happened. I offer my condolences to you. It was a shock to all of us. We never expected something like this to ever happen."

Liu bowed, but he did not like what the man's words implied. He was sure the monk was referring to Hua Yee and not Mr. Wu.

After a few minutes, they were ushered into the Abbot's office. He seemed surprised to see them. Liu took note of his reaction, but did not say anything. Pei Ke looked at Liu but said nothing either.

"Master Liu you have returned early from your trip to Beijing. We are all so sorry of course to hear about what happened to Wu and the children. It was so unfortunate what happened to Hua Yee."

Tears formed in Liu's eyes as he heard the words he feared the most. He heard Pei Ke stifle a groan, but he kept his attention on the Abbot. Liu knew that Pei Ke was just as heartbroken.

"Tell me exactly what happened. Where is Hua Yee?"

"We don't know a lot about what happened. One of the guards at Wu's place stumbled into town gravely wounded. He'd walked from Wu's compound and he collapsed when he got to the gates of the temple. We couldn't understand a lot of what he said, but we ascertained that someone had attacked Wu's place and that they needed help. We immediately contacted the local magistrate, and he and a few men went to Wu's place. I sent one of the monks along with them.

"When they returned, they gave a full report of the carnage that had taken place. There was no one alive when they arrived. I specifically asked about Hua Yee, but they said they hadn't seen her body among the dead. The guard who came to town died shortly after he arrived and could provide us no further useful information. He did tell us the attack started in the late evening hours while everyone was asleep. The attackers must have surprised the guards, and then attacked those within the compound."

"Who did this?" asked Liu as tears rolled down his cheeks. He could barely speak. He sat down and put his face in his hands. Pei Ke looked at his teacher and felt the pain Liu was suffering. He thought of Hua Yee and tears ran down his cheeks. The reality of what had happened had set in. There was to be no marriage between him and Hua Yee. With tears streaming down his cheeks, he looked at the Abbott and knew that the man had something to do with it.

He was about to ask when he realized it would be better for him to just listen. There just was too much killing taking place. There had to be an end to it. The more he thought about her, the angrier he became. He would do all he could to make Chen and his gang of thugs pay for this outrageous series of crimes they had committed against Liu's family. A void settled into his heart as a million thoughts went through his mind.

"We don't know," said the Abbot. "I asked the same question, and the men who went to Wu's compound did not know either. The assailants left no clues."

"What about Hua Yee?"

"When the men returned from Wu's I asked them about Hua Yee."

"Did they find her body?"

"She was not amongst the dead, at least according to the monk who accompanied them. Hua Yee was not there. They looked throughout the compound. Nobody knew where she was.

"The next morning I asked around the village if anyone had seen her. Everyone was shocked about what had happened, but no one had seen her. I then made the necessary Buddhist arrangements for the bodies to be buried at the Wu family gravesite. He did not have any known living relatives. His wife had died a few years ago. Quite a few men from the village, those who knew Wu, took care of the burial, and the guards were buried the next day.

"That same morning I had three monks go to your ancestral home in search of Hua Yee. I'm sad to say they found her on the mountain overlooking the valley. We can't know for sure what happened, but it appears the horse she was riding fell on top of her and trapped her beneath it. Her leg was broken, but she managed to crawl some distance before the cold overwhelmed her. The monks brought her body back to the temple and some of the ladies in the village prepared her body for burial."

He looked uncomfortable.

"We didn't know when you would return, and as you know, it is the custom here to bury the body as soon as possible. We went ahead and buried her and the other children at your ancestral gravesite next to her parents. We left a marker to identify the grave."

There is no need to worry," said Liu. "You did what was right. Was there any marks on her body that would suggest she'd been hurt or abused?"

"No. The women who prepared her would have told me. I only looked at the body when she was brought here. It is not appropriate for me to look at her uncovered body; that is for the women of the village to do.

"I think she must have been trying to go to your ancestral home to hide, which is too bad. If she had come here, maybe she would have been safe. We would have tried to protect her."

"Perhaps, but if she had come here, it may have simply led to more bloodshed. I don't think the attackers would have been stopped by a few Buddhist monks. Who took care of burying the children?"

"Even though the ground was frozen at the upper elevations where she died, it was not frozen in the valley and it was possible for us to bury them in your ancestral graveyard next to their parents."

"Was there any sign of violence to the horse?"

"No. I think it just lost its footing and fell on top of Hua Yee."

Liu shook his head sadly. Pei Ke looked at Liu and then at the Abbot. He was certain that the Abbot was not sharing some important information, but he had no way to challenge the Abbot.

"She was wearing the family amulet. Did you find it on her?" asked Liu.

"I wasn't aware she had it and as far as I know, she didn't have it when the monks found her."

"Did you ask them?"

"No, but I assumed they would have told me if they had found it. No mention was made of it by the ladies of the village."

As the two men talked, Pei Ke held back his emotions. He wanted to cry. He truly thought that Hua Yee would have made a wonderful wife. He had only known her for a short time, but tears were in his eyes. He would remember her for the rest of his life. Her death was just as senseless as the other deaths in the Liu family. His emotions turned from sadness to anger and back to sadness. He couldn't imagine what Liu was thinking at the moment. He was amazed his teacher could hold his composure under such circumstances.

"Where are you going now?" asked the Abbot.

"Is the boy here?"

"Yes, the servant boy is still with us and we are watching over him as you had instructed. We are taking care of him and teaching him as we teach all young boys who come to learn from us. Do you still want us to take care of him?"

"Yes, if you would. Where is he now?"

"He should be doing morning duties," said the Abbot

"I would like to see him."

The Abbot took Liu and Pei Ke into the large room where the boys were doing the daily sweeping and cleaning of the temple. Liu saw the boy off in the corner, sweeping around one of the statues.

"I would like to speak with him in private," Liu said to them. "Wait for me, and I will return in a few minutes."

Liu walked over to where the boy was sweeping.

"Good morning, Chang Song," said Liu.

The boy looked up in surprise and delight, then remembered to bow. Liu purposely stood in front of the boy to block the view of the Abbot and Pei Ke.

"How have you been?" asked Liu.

"Master, I'm fine. It is nice to see you again. I hear from the Abbot that more sadness has come to your family. I'm truly sorry this has happened to you. Are these the same men who killed your brother and my parents?"

"I am not sure, but I think so. As you know, one of them escaped when I rescued you. He probably wants revenge for the death of his father, and has taken it out on defenseless people who have never done anything to harm him.

"Has the Abbot and the other monks been treating you alright?"

"Yes and no. Sometimes the Abbot is mean. I really do not want to stay here much longer. I am not a monk and do not want to be a monk." He paused, then spoke quickly, like he was trying to get it all out. "Master, may I go with you and your student? I can be a servant to both of you, and you can teach me martial arts."

"Let me think about it for a little while. I need to make some plans. In the meantime, please stay here where it is safe and try to do as you are told. We can talk later.

"Now, your father was given an amulet by my family. He gave it to you to wear. Do you still have it?"

"Yes, I have it around my neck for safekeeping. It's really all I have of my parents and when I'm alone, I like to look at it." His face got serious. "But only when I'm alone. My father and mother told me to always safeguard it. They said your family gave it to them as a promise that someday we'd be rewarded for our many years of service."

"Has anyone ever asked you about it? Has anyone asked to see or touch it?"

"The Abbot asked me about it a couple of times. I just told him it was around my neck."

"Did he ever want to see it?"

"Yes, he asked to see it, but I had the feeling he was only curious about what it looked like. I gave it to him and he returned it a few days later."

Liu frowned. He felt very uneasy when he heard the Abbot had it for a couple of days. It might be possible to trace the outline of the amulet, even in a short time. With that and Hua Yee's piece, someone only needed to get one more piece of the amulet, and the shape of the fourth amulet could be determined.

Chang obviously noticed Liu's dark face and began to squirm.

"What does it matter if the Abbot sees it?" he asked.

Liu looked at him and put his hand on the boy's shoulder.

"You know you are to safeguard the amulet at all times. Do not let anyone see it or take it from you. What your parents told you is true. It is a key to a reward, but it is just one piece of the key. Others have other pieces and one day, you will all be together at one place and you can then show it to the others."

"Who else has one? Am I to just keep it around my neck as my parents wanted?"

"It is part of an ancient piece of metal work designed by my family. It is best you do not know who has the other pieces. There are three more, and I keep one of them."

They all look alike; however, there is a subtle difference between them. It is not important for you to know the difference. In fact, for your own safety it is best you only know that there are others and that one day the pieces will be brought together to form a whole. When that happens, you will be rewarded for keeping your part safe. Can I trust you to do everything in your power to keep the amulet safe and not give it to anyone who asks for it? Not even the Abbot?"

"Yes, Master. But how long do I have to stay here?"

"For now, it is best you learn as much as you can from the monks. I will speak to the Abbot to make sure he instructs you well. It is important you do well in your studies here. I know I can count on you to do your best."

"Master, my father told me you're very famous for your martial arts. Will you teach me one day?"

"We will see. For now, I trust you will do what I ask and study hard. Be the best you can be."

"Yes, Master. I will do my best. I will make you proud of me. I am forever grateful for what you have already done for me."

"I must go now and attend to some rather unpleasant duties."

The boy bowed low. Liu acknowledged him, then turned and walked back to where the Abbot and Pei Ke were standing. Liu motioned for them to walk. As they walked, they talked.

"Does the boy have any talent for studying?" asked Liu.

"Yes, he learns quickly," said the Abbot. "In fact, he learns faster than many of the other boys."

"Is there any way you can speed up the learning process for him?"

"We have a set method and curriculum we follow. Over generations, it's proven to be the correct way to teach. We teach age-appropriate material to all the boys. However, I might be able to have the monks spend some extra time with him, if you wish. Is there any particular material you want him to study?"

"Anything he excels in. In addition, I would like to make sure his legs become exceptionally strong. He needs to spend time in the horse stance."

"Is there a particular reason that you would like his legs to become strong?"

Liu stared at the Abbot but did not answer the question. Pei Ke was sure he knew.

"I will speak to the monks and see what can be done for the boy."

"I assume you have no financial requests from me?" asked Liu.

"No, Master, we are fine. We live the meager existence that is in keeping with our philosophy of purification. Your family in the past has been more than generous with us. This temple would not be here without the generosity of your family. The village supports our meager needs. When we are in need of something, we generally ask the villagers, and they collectively come to our aid. And, of course, your friend Mr. Wu has helped in the past."

Liu noticed that the Abbot looked uncomfortable.

"Master, what are you going to do now that you are back?"

"I need time to think through these recent developments. Have there been any outsiders in the village lately?"

"Not to my knowledge. Of course, we do not get involved with the daily activities of the villagers. We are here for their spiritual needs and not their secular ones."

Liu looked at the Abbot for a moment, absorbing what he had just said. Pei Ke was watching him too, pondering the whole conversation. He wanted to talk to his teacher in private.

"Master, do you and your student need to stay here at the temple? We have room for both of you for as long as you want. We would be honored to have you."

"Thank you, but we are going to go back to Wu's place to look around some more. Maybe there are some clues to help us determine who did this needless killing."

CHAPTER 32

Liu and Pei Ke said goodbye to the Abbot, walked out of his office, and immediately went to the statue of Kuan Yin. Liu felt someone was watching them while they prayed. As they bowed to the goddess, Liu took note of the large stones on the floor. He'd looked at them before. This time he saw scratches on one of the stones and he was certain that one or more of the stones had been moved.

After praying, they left the temple and turned toward the road leading to Mr. Wu's place. Riding down the road, Liu noticed one of the monks following them at a discrete distance. Once out of town, he stopped and turned to see if the man was still there, but the man was gone. Liu was not comforted by this.

"Master, I don't trust the Abbot."

"Why not?" asked Liu, turning to look at Pei Ke.

"He seems to be telling the truth, but I get the sense he isn't telling us everything. There's something he doesn't want us to know. I am sure of it."

"I had the same impression," said Liu. "He went out of his way to be convincing, but he tried a little too hard. That is why I told him we were going back to Wu's place. We are actually going to go my ancestral home and pay respect to my niece and the rest of the family who have died over this obsessive greed that exists within Chen."

"Maybe Chen and his men are there now. Should we get some men from the village to go with us?" His voice was harder than it was afraid.

"I do not think Chen wants to be discovered at either place. He has no business there and he'd have a lot of explaining to do if he was found there. Let us continue down this road for a few more minutes in case someone is watching us. Then we will be ride north to my ancestral home."

"Are we going back through the village?"

"No, we will circle around the village. It will take more time, but I do not want anyone to know I went north."

"You think the Abbot will tell everyone where you are going?"

"If the Abbot knows, then there is a good possibility someone else will know as well. I can think of no other reason for him to send one of the monks to follow us."

"Master, I do not trust the Abbot. I am not saying that he has done anything wrong, but he just seems to be distant during your conversations with him. It seems he is taking in information and then deciding what to do with the information. Do you trust him?"

"My grandfather and father have trusted the monks at the temple for many years, including the Abbot. He even has one of the pieces of the amulet, so clearly my father thought he was trustworthy."

"The amulet," Pei Ke said. The thought about all the time he'd worn it without knowing what it was.

Liu nodded.

"I know where three of the pieces are. I have one piece and it is the one that you are wearing. The Abbot has one, and so does the boy. But from what the Abbot told us, the one Hua Yee had is missing and I don't think she would have removed it on her own. Someone took it from her."

"You think the Abbot took it somehow? Was he involved in her death?"

"I hope not. I do not believe he would have willingly participated in that. I want to believe that he has no knowledge of where the amulet is, but I agree with you. He is hiding something. Did you notice that the stones in front of the statue of Kuan Yin had been moved?"

"No, Master, but what does that have to do with anything?"

Liu did not answer. Instead, he pointed to the side of the road where they were to lead the horses around the village.

CHAPTER 33

They guided their horses around the west side of the village to a point where it intersected with the road leading north toward Liu's ancestral home. Once on the road, they galloped part of the way, making up for the lost time. Riding up the side of the mountain, they came across the outline of the horse in the snow. There was not much left. The wild animals had had a feast.

Liu found a depression in the snow farther up the path, and assumed it was the place where Hua Yee had passed away. She was so close to her beloved valley. He stopped for a moment and said a little prayer to the Goddess of Mercy to guide Hua Yee in the afterlife. Tears formed as he stared at the indentation in the snow.

Pei Ke knelt down and touched the outline in the snow, and looked up at his master. No words needed to be exchanged between them, each felt the other's emotional turmoil. Liu looked around for any clues, but there was nothing in the snow that would help him resolve why this had happened.

At the crest of the mountain, they looked off into the valley. On the other side, there was snow, which diminished at the lower levels and disappeared in the valley. The difference in temperature between the crest of the mountain and the valley had to be at least thirty degrees.

Liu had always liked this view for the perspective it gave of the land, though it no longer looked the way he remembered it as a child. He wondered sadly, what he was going to do with the homes and the land, and his thoughts went back to Beijing and Ming Hong. What was she doing now with her son? Many things went through his mind. Things he should have done and things he should not have done. He had hated to leave Beijing so soon, but his highest priority was to get back here and resolve this problem with Chen.

They crossed over the crest and descended into the valley. Riding the horses downward, they felt the expected change in temperature. Pei Ke remembered the first time he'd ridden into the valley, the first time he'd seen Liu's ancestral home. The place had been covered by a pall of death. He couldn't imagine what his master was now feeling. Personally, he felt overwhelmingly sad. He couldn't get the thought of someone wanting to do harm to Hua Yee. The more he thought about it the angrier he became.

When they arrived at the main gate of Liu's ancestral home, they found it locked.

"Master, how do we get in if the gate is locked?"

"If the gate is locked that means it was locked from the inside."

"Maybe it is Chen and his men," said Pei Ke.

"It could be, but I do not think so. I think someone locked the gate and then jumped over the wall."

"Master, how are we going to get inside? The wall is over eight feet tall."

"We need to go to the west wall."

"Why the west wall?"

"These walls are covered with shards of broken glass and sharp pieces of metal. Anyone climbing over the wall would seriously cut their hands. However, there is one narrow part where there is no glass or metal.

"This four foot space is exactly fifteen feet from the southwest corner, and was established in case someone had to quickly climb the wall from the inside without cutting their hands. Follow me."

Liu rode around to the southwest wall and dismounted from his horse.

"Pei Ke guide your horse next to the wall, stand up on the saddle, and jump up to catch hold of the edge of the wall. Then pull yourself up and over."

Pei Ke looked at the wall and then at Liu.

"Master, this wall is almost eight feet tall. What if I miss?"

"Do not worry, you will not miss."

Pei Ke looked unconvinced and he stared nervously at his horse. Liu got down from his horse and walked over to them.

"I will hold on to the reins of the horse so he does not move. Go ahead."

Pei Ke took a deep breath, than stood carefully up on the saddle of the horse. Then without another word, he sprang up and grabbed the edge of the top of the wall.

"Good, now pull yourself up and over," said Liu.

Pei Ke did as instructed and was quickly on the ground on the other side of the wall. He looked carefully to see if there was anyone in the courtyard, but there was nothing out of the ordinary. He walked across the courtyard to the main gate, removed the heavy board locking the gate, and swung open the gate for Liu and the horses. Liu looked around just as Pei Ke had done, then pushed the gate closed and put the heavy timber in place, securing the gate from the inside.

They walked through the courtyard and then over to the living quarters and tied the horses to a tree near the house. They then walked around the immediate area looking for any evidence of foul play.

"Master, no one's here. Who locked the gate?"

"I do not know. It could have been Chen, as you said, or maybe the villagers who buried Hua Yee and the children. Maybe they wanted to make sure the compound was secure after seeing what happened at Mr. Wu's place."

"Do you think Chen will come here looking for you?"

"He has probably already been here and is now more than likely on his way back to Mr. Wu's place, hoping to find us there. Or, maybe I am wrong, and he feels he has nothing to lose by attacking us wherever he can find us. We must be on guard at all times."

He looked around thoughtfully.

"The more I think about it, the more I believe the Abbot is involved with all this. Maybe he became involved by chance or maybe he was coerced. Hopefully, I am wrong, but whatever happens, we will know soon. I am certain this will all play out in the next few days.

Let's look around."

Liu and Pei Ke walked around the inside of the compound, surveying each of the buildings. When the compound was originally built, there was only one structure, but as the extended family increased, more buildings were added to accommodate the additional inhabitants. Liu and Pei Ke studied the outside of each building. Testing a few doors and finding them locked.

"At least no one's been rummaging through things," said Pei Ke. Liu nodded.

They returned to the original building, which was the central focus in the compound, and was where Liu had grown up as a child. It was also the place Hua Yee would have called home.

Here, they found the door unlocked and Liu immediately knew someone had been here since he'd left. The table and chairs were moved and some of the other furniture was not quite where he remembered it to be.

"Pei Ke, someone has been here and I do not think it was the villagers. They would have no reason to come into this building. Whoever came here took pains to cover their tracks, so I doubt it was crooks who came to steal. It had to be someone who had an interest in keeping the property in decent order. It had to be Chen and his men."

"Master, did they take anything?"

"I do not think so, but we will look in all the rooms to make sure nothing is missing."

They walked together from the main sitting room down the hallway to Hua Yee's room. As they walked into the room, Liu saw a piece of rice paper on her bed. Liu picked it up and looked at it for a few moments. He gazed upward in thought.

"Master, what does it say?"

Liu gave it to Pei Ke, who read the contents carefully.

> *Liu, you've stolen this land, which is rightfully mine.*
> *I know you will be reading this soon. When you finish*
> *reading it, you will know you have little time to live.*

"Master, there is no signature on this paper. Do you think Chen wrote it?" said Pei Ke. Liu nodded.

"There is no doubt in my mind he wrote it. He still has greed and deceitfulness in his heart, which I think will never go away. It is impossible to reason with such a person. No matter what I would tell him he would not believe it. I see only two solutions to this problem, neither one of which I care to entertain.

"Pei Ke, we need to be extremely vigilant. He will have his men everywhere looking for us. I think we are safe here tonight, but after tonight, we will need to leave. When there is an altercation between us, I want it to be of the time and place of my choosing, not his. That means we need to surprise him and not allow him to surprise us. I am going to rely on you to help as much as possible when the time comes. If you feel anger, try to suppress it and rely only on your training so you do not make costly mistakes."

Pei Ke looked at Liu and nodded.

"Master you can count on me."

"Pei Ke, I want to go out to the graveyard and pay respect to my family and ancestors. Would you like to join me?"

"Yes, Master. To be honest, after all that's happened, I feel I am part of your family and I would like to pay my respects to your family, and especially to Hua Yee. She had a special place in my heart and I want to tell her that. I looked forward to coming back here and I was going to talk to you about her."

"Yes, I know she was special to you. Uncle Wu mentioned he thought there was a mutual attraction between you two, of which I would have approved. Of course, I would have approved of another union if that had been your choice. That is why I want you to be with me when I visit the graves. I want you to understand you have a special place in my heart."

Pei Ke looked at Liu and again nodded. He did not know what to say.

"Master," Pei Ke said softly, "I would be honored to visit the graves with you and pay respect to your ancestors."

"Before we go, I would like to accept you into the family as an inner door student to carry on the tradition of my teachings. You will join in with a few other students, who also have been accepted into the family. Wei Ken De is one of them, and there are others, who you do not know. Maybe one day you will have the opportunity to meet them. They are now very accomplished martial artists."

"Master I am honored to be accepted into your family. I will do honor to you and your family and will uphold the Liu family traditions."

Liu led Pei Ke back to the main sitting room and had him kneel down in front of a statue of Kuan Yin.

"Pei Ke, repeat these words."

Pei Ke repeated the words that solidified him within the Liu clan. He felt honored to be one of the few that would carry on the traditions of the Liu family martial art teachings. He was overwhelmed, but his tears were of joy rather than sadness.

"Master, I will be loyal to you and your family for the rest of my life. I will carry on the traditions as you have taught them to me."

Pei Ke bowed low to Liu, and Liu acknowledged the respect paid to him.

"Even though you are now an inner door student studying from me, you must remember your place amongst those who have gone before you. They have the experience and the training, which has carried them to where they are now. Learn from them and do so with humility and honor. Never let your ego prevent you from moving forward. You have talent and the ability that many do not have. You have learned how to learn, which is an ability that is not teachable. Students either have it or they don't. Never disgrace what you have come to be a part of today."

Liu motioned for Pei Ke to follow him, and they went out the main gate to the Liu family graveyard. The burial site was to the east, between the outer walls of the compound and a nearby forest. The burial site was chosen by Liu's grandfather so that the inhabitants of the graveyard could see and feel the energy of the rising sun.

Pei Ke followed Liu as he walked to the fresh graves. There were identifying marks on the freshly turned ground. Liu knelt in front of Hua Yee's grave and bowed three times. Pei Ke followed and listened to the words of Liu as he prayed to Kuan Yin to look after the spirits of Hua Yee and the children.

Still kneeling, Liu looked to the heavens and stretched out his arms. Pei Ke stretched out his own arms, and as he did, he could feel the Universal Energy flowing not only into himself, but into his teacher as well. He was becoming more in tune with his teacher, and for a brief moment he thought that he was becoming part of his teacher's energy. He was merging into what his teacher was and it felt good. He wanted more of it.

He closed his eyes and prayed on his own to Kuan Yin to give him the guidance to do what he needed to do in life to make sure he was a credit to the Liu family. He prayed to Hua Yee and promised her she would always have a special place in his heart no matter what happened in his life. He was sorry her life had ended so soon and he believed the Universal Energy would always be there for the two of them. He told her he would avenge her death and the death of all those within the Liu family who died at the hands of the Chen family. He would gladly give his life to take revenge. In no way would her death and the death of those before her go without retribution. Though he knew the odds against them were high, he said these things with calm certainty.

Liu and Pei Ke prayed for ten more minutes. Each shared their thoughts with the departed ones and the Universal Energy. Pei Ke had no idea what Liu was praying about, but had a good idea it was similar to what he had prayed. He felt very close to his teacher, closer than he had ever felt before. Liu was now more than just a teacher, and there was more than just a teacher-student relationship. There was a bond that would never be broken, and he was entwined within the events unfolding for both of them.

Liu bent forward and touched his head to the ground three times. Pei Ke followed suit and then stood as Liu rose to his feet. They both turned and walked back towards the main gate. They entered the compound in silence, each deep in thought. Liu thought of his childhood, and how wonderful it had been. One thought after the other flooded through his mind. Each thought preceded by the realization that his family was dead and if he would have been there, he might have prevented it.

Pei Ke thought of Hua Yee, and how a beautiful girl's life had been cut short by the evil actions and hatred of one man. Even though Chen had not killed her, her death had forever changed his life.

"Pei Ke, we are going to stay here for the night. Look around the rooms including the servants quarters and see if you see anything unusual."

"Master, what are you going to do?"

"I am going to sit here and just meditate for a while. I need to calm my mind and spirit and prepare myself for what is to come."

"May I sit with you?"

"Another time."

Pei Ke walked off and Liu sat upright in his chair. He wanted to communicate with the Universal Energy and he did not want to be disturbed by questions or any other energy fields. He calmed his mind and made the necessary energy connections to the Yin energy of the earth and the Yang energy of the heavens. He called upon the forces of nature to help him visualize what was now taking place in the vast sphere of energy that surrounded him.

He focused on his breath and meditated for over an hour. His diligence was rewarded with an instant clear picture in his mind of Chen and his men arguing over what to do next. They were several miles away, hidden on a plateau overlooking a small creek south of Wu's place.

Liu had never been to the place, but he knew how to get there. This did not surprise him. He had experienced many strange things while meditating. When he was in such a state he could see what others could not see, he could smell what others could not smell, and he could hear what others could not hear. Even though he could do all these things, he was still aware of his current surroundings as he sat on the chair at his ancestral home. He noticed Pei Ke coming into the room and watched him for a few minutes before he went off to some other area of the house, but this did not disturb his state of mind.

He listened as Chen's men argued. He counted ten or more of them not including Chen himself. Liu processed the information and then returned his consciousness to his own surroundings. The Universal Energy had provided him with enough information to defeat Chen and his men.

Pei Ke walked back into the room and saw Liu sitting quietly.

"Master, I did not want to disturb you before. I looked all around this part of the house and the servant's quarters and I did not find anything unusual or out of place."

"Chen was here at least once and maybe twice. I do not think he will return tonight. We need to get some sleep. Take the third room on the right down the hallway. It was Hua Yee's room. I am going to sleep in my old bedroom."

"Yes, Master. Should one of us be on guard?"

"I do not think so. It is late and we need to get some sleep."

"Master, is there anything I can do for you before I go to sleep?"

"No."

Pei Ke wanted to say something, but he wasn't sure exactly what, so he simply bowed and walked to Hua Yee's room. He felt the energy in his body change as he passed through the doorway. He gently closed the door and walked over to the bed. He looked at the bed, and sensed she was in the room waiting for him.

Lying in bed Pei Ke thought of Hua Yee. She was so beautiful. She definitely would have made a fine wife in all the classical traditions of a Chinese family. What a waste for a life to end so soon. He sensed she was lying next to him. He could feel her energy. He wanted to be part of that energy. He wanted her. A small tear formed in his eye as he fell asleep thinking about her as his wife.

Liu lay in his own bed thinking about not only the tragic waste of his niece's life, but the tragic waste of the rest of his family. Why would someone go to the lengths Chen and his father had resorted to in order to obtain this land? He fell asleep, but it was fitful. Possibilities and scenarios went through his head; some of them passed through his mind more than once.

He woke up several times in a cold sweat. He looked around the room. It was the room he had slept in as a child; and now it was the room he was sleeping in as an adult. Each time he woke up, he longed to be able to go back to the days of his childhood. He remembered his mother reading to him at night after he had changed into his night clothes. No matter how tired she was, she would lay next to him and read him stories from the classic works of Chinese literature. He'd remembered those stories all his life.

They stayed at Liu's ancestral home for two days. They explored the remaining buildings again and still found nothing unusual. Liu took Pei Ke to boundary markers delineating the full extent of the property handed down through decades. Each boundary marker had the name of the Liu family chiseled on it. In all instances, it was a huge boulder buried in the ground. It would be almost impossible for anyone to move the boulder and if anyone were to destroy the chiseled name on the boulder, it would be obvious to whoever looked that something had been written there.

CHAPTER 34

L iu and Pei Ke rose before dawn and did their Qi Gong in the courtyard. After practicing, they went to the gravesite and paid their respect again to the Liu family.

"Pei Ke let's pray in silence to Kuan Yin. We both need to ask her for guidance."

Pei Ke reiterated what he had said two nights before, promising to Hua Yee and the ancestors of the Liu family that he, as an adopted member of the family, would do his duty to avenge them.

After, Pei Ke closed and locked the gate and once again scaled the back wall. The two of them rode away from the compound. They slowly made their way to the crest of the mountain. As they rode over the crest, they both turned and looked back into the valley. Pei Ke once again marveled at its beauty. There was sadness in what he was leaving. He did not know when or if he would ever be returning to Liu's ancestral home.

Descending along the path, Liu stopped his horse and looked to his right. He sensed that eyes were following him but they were not close. Rather, they were somewhere off in the distance. He looked at Pei Ke, and this time, he knew his student sensed them too. Pei Ke pointed in the direction where Liu was looking and Liu nodded and then urged his horse forward.

He was getting very tired of those eyes and the evilness they represented.

CHAPTER 35

They rode into the village and went directly to the temple to pray. As they entered, one of the monks approached them.

"Master Liu, the Abbot would like to see you," said the monk somewhat sheepishly.

"Can it wait for a few minutes so that we can pray?"

"The Abbot indicated it was important to see you immediately."

Liu and Pei Ke glanced at each other, but went with the monk to the Abbot's office and were immediately shown in to see him. Liu looked at the Abbot's ashen face and knew something was amiss.

"Master Liu, I don't know how to tell you this but the boy is dead."

"What? What happened to him?" asked Liu.

Pei Ke saw that all the color went out of Liu's face and his shoulders seemed to drop as an additional burden had been thrust upon him.

"We do not know what actually happened," answered the Abbot. "The monks sent him to the creek to draw water, but he never returned. When the monks realized he was gone too long, they went looking for him. They found him a little ways from the creek. The water buckets were full but they were still in the creek."

"What happened to him? Did you yourself go looking for him?"

"No. I did not know he was missing until I was told about it from the others who went looking for him. They brought his body back to the temple and called me. I immediately went to see the body when they called me. It is always distressing when a member of the temple passes away. In this case it is even more distressing because he was brutally murdered."

"Why would anyone want to kill a young boy? He never did anything to anyone. Do you know of anyone that could possibly be involved in this heinous act?"

Pei Ke watched the Abbot's face as he formulated an answer. The Abbot cast his eyes down slightly as he replied. Pei Ke immediately knew there was no longer any doubt whatsoever that the Abbot was somehow involved in the ongoing attacks against the Liu family. If there was an attack against the Liu family then there was an attack against him. Pei Ke looked at Liu and he could see the anger whelming up in his teacher. Pei Ke wondered how Liu could control his emotions to that extent knowing that the Abbot was surely involved with what had happened.

"From what I could discern, he was beaten to death. There were bruises on his body and head, indicative of being struck by some type of a blunt object like a club."

"How do you know it was a club?" asked Liu.

Pei Ke looked at the Abbot and could see a faint feeling of uneasiness in the Abbot's demeanor. Pei Ke looked at Liu but Liu did not change his expression. The Abbot hesitated for a fraction of a second as he peered into Liu's eyes. Then he responded.

"I do not know if it was a club. I am only guessing by the bruises on his body. There were marks on his head and other parts of his body."

"When was he killed?" asked Liu.

"He was found dead the same day you left here. We buried him yesterday in the temple cemetery according to our customs. I led the prayer ceremony, as is the custom at this temple. The rest of the monks attended the funeral. In our tradition, it is a simple ceremony. He has passed on from this life to another and hopefully he will be at peace with his new life."

"I think he should have been buried with his parents at my ancestral home. Why did you bury him so quickly after his death?"

"He is a student here, and it has always been the custom to bury any member of the temple in our own graveyard. We take care of the gravesite and regularly have devotions to those who have gone before us."

"You have part of the amulet my father gave you. The boy also had one. Did you find it on his body when you prepared him for burial?"

"No," said the Abbot. "There was nothing on his body except his clothes."

Liu looked hard at the Abbot trying to discern the truth of the Abbot's statement. He could see the Abbot's left eye twitch. He knew that the Abbot was lying. His first instinct was to confront the Abbot with all the evidence he had, but realized that might not be wise at this moment.

"Did you make any inquires in the community about what happened?"

"We asked around, but no one knew or heard anything."

"You still have your part of the amulet?"

"Of course," said the Abbot. "It has been in my possession ever since your father gave it to me for safekeeping."

"Hua Yee is also dead. Doesn't that seem strange to you that two people associated with me are now dead?"

"Yes." The Abbot spoke stiffly, evasively. "As I told you before, we discovered her body and had her remains buried at your parents cemetery."

"She also had a piece of the coin, but as we discussed before, it is also missing."

"You and I are the only two who wear our amulets legitimately."

Pei Ke looked at the Abbot and again instinctively knew that the Abbot was not telling the truth. He could not decide if the Abbot was outright lying or simply omitting some significant piece of information. Did he have the two amulets? Had he had the boy killed? Pei Ke hoped that Liu could see through the subterfuge. He debated whether or not he should somehow bring it up.

"I suspect the amulets are forever lost," said the Abbot. "If someone does turn up with them, we know he is an imposter and that he committed a crime to get them, they found them, or someone gave it to them. Maybe we should distribute the estate of your parents as indicated by your father. Since there are only two of us, the split would be one fourth to you and one fourth to the temple for guarding the fortune. The other two parts are for the distribution to the poor. I will take charge of making sure that the poor get whatever needs to be distributed."

No sooner had the words left the Abbot's mouth then Liu felt an uneasiness within the Universal Energy. Liu sensed Pei Ke had felt the same thing and looked at his student. No words were exchanged, but they both knew at that precise moment that the Abbot was positively and intimately involved in whatever had happened to the boy and possibly to Hua Yee. Liu looked at the Abbot for a moment, searching for the appropriate words. He was about to speak when Pei Ke interrupted.

"Master, maybe we should.."

"Pei Ke, please. I know you are hungry, but we can eat later. Right now, I want to pray to Kuan Yin. I have always found solitude in praying to her."

Pei Ke was initially caught off guard by the statement, but quickly realized that Liu had in a very subtle way, told him to keep his mouth shut.

"Yes, Master."

"I would like to go and pray now. Would you please excuse us?"

Liu gave a short bow to the Abbot and turned.

"Of course," said the Abbot.

Liu and Pei Ke walked out of the Abbot's office. Neither one of them looked back, but they both felt the eyes of the Abbot on them as they walked down the hallway towards the main devotional area. When they were out of hearing range from the Abbot, Liu took his arm and placed it on Pei Ke's shoulders as they walked.

"First of all, how many times have I told you not to interrupt me when I am talking?"

"I am truly sorry, Master. It was just..." Pei Ke hesitated and then spoke. "I wanted somehow to warm you we should discuss some things before you committed yourself to anything."

"Pei Ke, how long have you been my student?"

"Master, it has been some time now."

"Don't you think that I am aware of what is happening with the Abbot? His statements are not truthful. He knows more than he is telling me and I need to find out what is happening. I am certain that he has directly or indirectly been involved in the death of the boy and Hua Yee."

"Yes, Master," Pei Ke said sheepishly. "Of course, Master. And I agree with you. He is not being truthful and I did not want you to say something which would commit you to something with him. In my opinion, he is not to be trusted. I am trying to do my duties to look after the Liu family name."

"I agree. The second thing is that I see that you have again sensed a disruption in the Universal Energy."

"Master, was that what I sensed when we crossed over the mountain to come here and when I realized he was lying to us?"

"It is part of it. It is coming to rely on your own energy to guide you in whatever you do. Cultivate it from now on. Come to appreciate what it can do for you in your future journeys, whatever and wherever they may be."

"Master, what are we going to do now?"

"We are going to pray to Kuan Yin and then we are going to go to the gravesite of the boy and pay our respects to him. His family has been faithful to my family for many years, and the least I can do is to pay my respects. As far as I know, there are no other survivors in his family. After that I will decide on what to do."

After praying to Kuan Yin, Liu and Pei Ke walked to the graveyard behind the temple. It was easy to find the grave. The ground had been disturbed and there was a small marker with the appropriate name on it. Liu bowed at the gravesite and Pei Ke followed his lead in paying respect. Liu promised the boy that he would find out who had done this and take appropriate revenge.

CHAPTER 36

Liu and Pei Ke walked away from the temple, purposely leaving their horses tethered to a tree. They walked through the village and headed down a side street. Liu recognized some of the villagers and greeted them with a slight nod of his head.

"Master, where are we going?"

"We are going to get something to eat before we leave the village. There is a little place I know where they have excellent Do Jiang and Shao Bing Yue Tiao. I also need to think for a few minutes. I left the horses at the temple so the Abbot would know I am still in the village."

"Master, have you eaten here before?"

"I first came here when I was a child. The small restaurant has been handed down within the family for two generations. Everyone knows that the owner serves the best food in the village. I know the current owner. Since many people in the village come to his restaurant, he might have an insight into what is happening."

The restaurant was in the middle of the block, and there was a very small, nondescript sign over its door. It was one of those places you needed to know where to go to get to it, but everyone in the village knew where it was.

The restaurant was not large, having only ten tables, and due to the time of the morning, it was virtually empty except for a lone couple sitting at one of the tables. Pei Ke could smell the wonderful fragrance of soybean milk as they entered. Liu and Pei Ke walked to the back of the restaurant and took a table in one of the corners.

"Master Liu, welcome once again," said the restaurant owner as he bustled over to them. "I haven't seen you in some time. I would like to offer my condolences for your loss. We have known your family for many years, and it is always a shock when you hear about such tragedy. If there is anything that I can do to help you, please let me know. If those men are ever caught they should be hanged immediately."

"Thank you," said Liu

"What would you like today?"

"This is my student Pei Ke."

Pei Ke bowed in respect to an elder, and the restaurant owner just smiled and turned to Liu.

"We would like some Do Jiang, some Shao Bing Yue Tiao, and some of your nice tasting tea."

"You have remembered about my tea."

"Yes, I understand that you harvest it on your own farm up in the mountains and prepare it right here in your restaurant."

"Yes. As far as I know, it is the finest tea within hundreds of miles. Of course, I am quite modest about it."

Liu laughed and motioned for the owner to sit with them.

"You are conversant with what happens here in the village and you know that misfortune has befallen my family more than once. Have you heard anything that you think I should be aware of?"

"There was a period of time when we had some strangers come through the village. They purchased supplies and from what I heard, they camped out near your ancestral home. This was about the time your parents were killed. Well, everyone in the village knows you took care of them. However, it seems within the last week or so another group has come through the village and they have purchased some supplies. They keep to themselves, but they did eat here recently."

"Did any of them spend any time praying at the temple?"

"As a matter of fact they did. A couple of times when I was closing for the evening, I would walk out to the main street and see one or two strange horses at the temple. I know it seems odd I would mention these horses, but their horses were not farm animals, but appeared to be riding horses, which is why I noticed. You can tell the difference between a work horse and a riding horse, and these were definitely riding horses."

"Did you see the men yourself?"

"No, but there were only two horses so I guess there were only two men. "The whole village was shocked to hear what has been happening to your family and also to Mr. Wu. He was a friend of mine, just like your brother was a friend. Whoever did these evil deeds needs to be punished."

He stood up.

"I'll go get your food. Everything is on me today."

"That is not necessary."

"I insist."

Liu bowed and the owner left to prepare the food.

"Master, just because he only saw two horses doesn't mean there aren't more men. They could have been hiding in the forest or on one of the many mountains in this area. Chen could have his men dispersed to numerous locations so that we cannot find him."

"Yes, I know. I suspect he has ten or more men with him now."

"Where does he get these men? Did they come from this area or did he bring them with him when he came?"

"I do not think any of his men came from here. If they had come from this area, sooner or later, they would have been recognized by some of the villagers. There are always men willing to compromise their values for some gain, and there are men who are always deceived into thinking they can get away with the most heinous of crimes without any retribution."

Liu and Pei Ke waited for the restaurant owner to return with their breakfast. Each was contemplating the events that may or may not take place in the next couple of days. When their breakfast arrived, they ate in silence. While Pei Ke was finishing his tea, Liu rose and walked over to the owner. Liu motioned for Pei Ke to stay seated. Liu and the restaurant owner walked to the rear of the restaurant. Liu came back ten minutes later holding a piece of folded rice paper.

"Pei Ke, hold on to this for me. I will explain later."

Pei Ke took the folded rice paper and put it inside his shirt. Liu sat down and Pei Ke poured his teacher some more tea.

"Master, this tea really is good. It is equivalent to the tea we had when we first started this journey some time ago."

"I agree, this is good tea. It would be nice for us to just sit here and have a relaxing conversation, but we must go."

Liu stood up and Pei Ke followed. Liu thanked the owner for the breakfast, and the two of them walked outside.

CHAPTER 37

They retraced their steps back through the alley to the temple. Approaching the temple, Liu and Pei Ke could see the monks making some minor repairs on the façade of the building. Liu nodded to the monks and the monks out of courtesy returned the greeting. Liu and Pei Ke mounted their horses and rode out of town north toward Liu's ancestral home. When they were a little more than a mile out of town, and Liu was certain they were not being followed, he told Pei Ke.

"Pei Ke, I want you to circumvent the village like we did before, then ride south to see Wei Ken De. Deliver the note I gave to you. It should be given to him and him alone. As we discussed before, I would like him to join us in taking care of Chen and his men. You and I are too outnumbered to do it ourselves. He needs to come quickly and help us. Explain the details to him and Mei Li."

"What will you be doing?"

"Let me finish first. When the two of you return, meet me at Wu's place. On horseback, it shouldn't take you too long. If I am not there, just wait for me."

"What will you be doing while I am gone?"

"I am going to go see the elders in the village we stayed in on our way back from Beijing. You remember they hired the three Hu brothers to protect their village? I am going to see if they will help us as well. If so, then this coming altercation will be evenly matched. I think I can be back by the same time you arrive. I will meet you at Wu's."

He looked at Pei Ke for a moment, than said.

"I want you to go now and be vigilant as to your surroundings. I need you back in one piece."

"Right now?"

"Yes, and do not lose my sack."

Pei Ke nodded, then turned and started to head south toward the village.

"Pei Ke, be sure to skirt around the village, and do not go through it, and be sure and safeguard the sack that you are carrying."

"Yes, Master."

Pei Ke hurried off and Liu left for the village to the east. He trusted Pei Ke would be able to do what was asked of him. It would be the first time he had asked Pei Ke to go off on his own. Hopefully, he would be up to the challenge. Once he got to Wei Ken De's place there would be no problem.

CHAPTER 38

Chen was getting feedback on a haphazardly basis. Some of it was confusing and contradictory, but he felt this latest piece of information about Liu was accurate enough for him to act on immediately. He had been camped west and south of Wu's place, off the main roads in a rural forest area isolated from the rest of the countryside. He did not want his whereabouts to be known, and he wanted to choose the time of his action rather than have Liu choose it for him.

The latest information was that Liu and his awkward student, were headed north from the village to Liu's ancestral compound. He would give Liu plenty of time to get there and then he could attack that night and finally wipe the old man out. Once the deed was done, he could go back to Beijing and claim the valley and the surrounding lands as his own.

Gaining access to the Liu compound would be easy, as he discovered the one unprotected area on the wall. It was an old idea that had been passed down forever. He would take his men and camp out in the mountains near the valley. They would enter the compound in the middle of the night when both Liu and his student were asleep. It would be fast and effective. He smiled as he gathered his men to head north. He first had to get to the road leading from Wu's place to the village and then head north through the village to Liu's place.

He sent two men ahead of them to scout the way and make sure there were no surprises. Chen hated surprises. He gave the men strict orders. If they saw something unusual, they were not to get involved. They were to ride back and report to him and he would decide what to do.

CHAPTER 39

Pei Ke skirted around the village as Liu had directed. Once past the village, he headed south along the same road he and Liu had taken before.

Chen was headed east to meet up with the south road which was to take him north past Wu's place and through the village.

Liu headed east away from the village traveling toward Beijing and the elders of the village where they had twice stayed.

Little did Liu know that Pei Ke was heading into imminent danger and the ultimate test of his abilities in martial arts. If he had known, he never would have sent Pei Ke south to see Wei Ken De.

CHAPTER 40

Riding away from the village, Liu came to the split in the road. He looked to the left and then to the right. It seemed like it was only a short time ago that he was at this spot. The last time he was here, he took the road to the left. This time he took the branch to the right. He knew there were more travelers on this road, but it was faster of the two routes and he had no time to enjoy the journey. His life and the lives of others depended on him getting to his destination as fast as possible.

He hoped the Hu brothers were still at the village and that they would be willing to help him. If not, then he would have to deal with Chen and his men another way. Either way, Liu knew this must be the end of the continual battle between them. He planned to win and he expected the Universal Energy to help him in his efforts.

He thought briefly of Pei Ke, hoping the boy would remember all he'd learned, then turned his attention to his own task. He remembered the last time he had made this journey; he had taken the other road, expecting a leisurely trip. Soon after, he'd been accosted by those evil eyes that had been following him. There were no such eyes now.

The road to the right would take him south of where he wanted to go, but he knew there was a way to head north to his destination once he got in the general area of the village. He was thankful the horse he was riding had lasted this long.

CHAPTER 41

The two men Chen sent ahead reached the main north south road and headed north toward the village. They had been recruited by Chen in one of the outlying areas just west of Beijing, and were promised that they would be able to get a portion of Chen's inheritance and family fortune if they could kill Liu. They would be doing everyone a favor and would forever gain the appreciation of Chen, who was the rightful owner of the land and its fortune.

They had seen the document Chen had, granting the land to his father. There were other men in the group, who indicated Chen had been to the emperor's office to have the document legitimized. Based on this information, they felt that they were doing Chen a favor. Regardless, they wanted to share in the Liu fortune, and were willing to kill to get it.

CHAPTER 42

Pei Ke pushed his horse hard once he circumvented the village. He was determined to get to Wei Ken De's place as soon as possible and explain to Liu's senior student what had taken place. He felt honored that Liu had asked him to do this. He felt even more honored that Liu had entrusted him again with the amulet. He wondered why Liu just did not take what he wanted from the Abbot.

The amulets were nice. He had been given an explanation as to their importance. But he did not fully understand the significance; however, he would safeguard it around his neck until death, as well as the sack he was carrying. He knew the sack contained information that was valuable to Liu, and there were other secrets in it that only Liu could explain.

Suddenly, Pei Ke saw the two men ahead of him. They were riding quite leisurely along the road as if they were simply two men out for a ride. A sense of uneasiness came over him, which he could not identify. Pei Ke did not yet have Liu's ability to immediately sense evilness and danger, and thus he rode to within fifty feet of the men before one of them suddenly recognized him.

"That's Liu's partner shouted one of the men. Let's get him."

"I thought we were only supposed to observe and report back to Chen," said the second man.

"Forget it said the first rider."

Pei Ke was caught completely off guard as the men galloped towards him. They closed the distance swiftly. One of men grabbed the reins from Pei Ke's hands. Without thinking, Pei Ke leaped from his horse onto the assailant's horse. They struggled awkwardly for a moment. The horse became frightened and reared up, throwing both men to the ground. By the time Pei Ke could get up, the man was already on his feet and deftly grabbed Pei Ke's wrist. Pei Ke struggled to break the hold, but the man was just too strong.

A voice in the back of his head told him to relax and drop his elbow. As he dropped his elbow below the level of his wrist, he could feel the structure of his body change and he was now in command. He utilized one of the Chin Na moves that Liu had taught him and dislocated the bones in the man's wrist. While the man was withering on the ground, Pei Ke saw out of the corner of his eye that the assailant's partner was dismounting.

While still holding on to the first man's wrist, Pei Ke's mind flashed back to the promise to protect the Liu family name and avenge the cruel death of Liu's family. He thought of Hua Yee, the beautiful Hua Yee, who had died because of the actions of Chen. With a quick downward strike of his foot, Pei Ke broke the man's neck. Pei Ke heard it snap and there was no remorse in his heart. The man would have killed him and he had done what he had to do.

The second man ran toward Pei Ke with an evil grin on his face. As he approached, he drew out his broadsword and began to swing it back and forth. When the man was within five feet, Pei Ke stepped left into the back part of the arc of the broad sword as it swung past his body. The sword missed him by no more than a couple of inches.

Pei Ke grabbed the man's right hand with his own right hand and held on tightly. With his left forearm, Pei Ke brought it forcefully down on the inside of the man's elbow. He remembered what Liu had drilled into him many times before; a rotating surface always worked better than a non-rotating surface. As Pei Ke rotated his forearm against the man's inside elbow crease, the man's arm easily bent causing the broadsword to arc upwards. Pei Ke then pushed the man's right hand and the broadsword sliced across the man's neck. Blood squirted as the man collapsed and gasped curses at Pei Ke. Pei Ke just watched the man jerk and wither for a couple of minutes. The color went from his face and cheeks as he bled out. Pei Ke wasted no time in dragging both men away from the road and hiding their bodies behind some fallen trees.

He then took their horses into the forest where they could not be seen from the road and tied their reins to a low hanging branch. After covering the bloodstains on the road, as best he could with dirt from the side of the road, he led his own horse into the forest.

He sat down, put his face into his hands, and cried. The tears turned into sobs. He must have cried for ten minutes. His thoughts rationalized his actions. Deep down he was happy they were dead. It was either them or him, and he had vowed to avenge Hua Yee's death. The Universal Energy would understand.

He sat there for over an hour contemplating what he had done when he heard horses trotting up the road from the south. He stealthily moved toward the road to get a better view. He was too far away to make out exactly who it was but he was sure that it was Chen and his men. He debated whether or not to go find his teacher but thought better of the idea. He needed to get to Wei Ken De. He walked back to his horse and sat back down on the cold ground and listened to the hoofs moving off into the distance. When they were gone, he got up, walked over to the two dead men and spit on their bodies. He took the reins of his horse, and walked to the road. He looked northward up the road but could see no one. If it was Chen and his men, they were not in a hurry. He mounted his horse and continued on his journey south to see Wei Ken De.

CHAPTER 43

Liu patted the horse's neck and urged him forward. He wanted the horse to run at a full gallop all the way, but he knew that the horse did not have the stamina. He would just have to judge the condition of the road and what the horse could tolerate.

The last time he headed to Beijing, he had experienced the evil eyes. This time they were nowhere to be seen or felt. He thought about that fact for a few minutes, but discounted that it really meant anything.

One day later, he rode into the village. It was dark as he entered the village. It was not more than a couple of minutes until he was again met by the Hu brothers. As they rode up, the brothers recognized him and nodded. Liu returned the greeting and started to speak, but the three men turned and indicated he should follow them. The four of them passed through the center of the village and stopped at a familiar house. As Liu dismounted, the Hu brothers rode on to where they were staying. A door opened and one of the village elders stood in the doorway. After a few seconds, he recognized Liu and greeted him.

"Master Liu, you have returned. What a wonderful surprise. We did not expect you back so soon. Where is Pei Ke? Is he coming with you?"

"I have come by myself, and I need to speak with you. I have a favor to ask. May I come in? I know it is late."

"Of course, come in. It is never too late for you."

Liu walked into the elder's home and followed the man into the kitchen. He sat down as the elder poured some hot water into the teapot.

"It is so good to see you once again. The villagers talk about you every day. I think they expect one day you will ride into our village and stay permanently. They will be surprised to see you back so soon."

"Once again, I'm afraid I will not be here long. Maybe not even the night. I need your help. But let me explain to you what has happened."

Liu went on to explain what had happened during the last few months. He shared with the elder the fight on the mountain with the Chen family and his trip to Beijing when he had first came through the village. He indicated the younger Chen had amassed a group of approximately ten or more men and their objective was to kill him and get title to the Liu family ancestral lands. He could not fight them by himself and needed help from some professional martial artists.

"Master Liu, I assume you are asking if the men guarding our village can come to your aid?"

"Yes."

"As far as I'm concerned, there's not a problem with it, but it is not for me to say. The Hu brothers guard the village for us and we pay them, and I do not know if they would agree to do it for you. Also, the villagers need to have a say, since they are paying the guards, and we have to consider that the guards will not be here to protect us. I don't think we'd have a problem, but we never know.

"What we need to do is have you first talk with the Hu brothers and see if they're willing to help you. If they won't help, then it would be no use for us to approach the villagers. It is late and you have come a long way. The place where you and Pei Ke stayed is still vacant. I will take you there and you can sleep there for the night. In the morning, we can discuss the situation with the brothers and then with the elders of the village."

That night Liu stayed up for a couple of hours, reviewing in his mind the sequence of events that had taken place. He was optimistic about what was coming. He wondered if Pei Ke had reached Wei Ken De's place yet.

CHAPTER 44

L iu woke early, as was his custom. He looked out the window and saw a dusting of snow on the ground. It was late winter now and early spring would be just a few short weeks away. Soon the leaves would be showing and a new season of life would blossom on the land. Liu looked forward to the spring. Hopefully, this year the spring would bring a time without conflict.

Liu was once more deep in thought when he heard a soft knock on the door. Opening the door, he saw not only the elders of the village, but also many of the villagers. He recognized some of them from his visits before. They all started to clap and Liu smiled and bowed in recognition. Behind the crowd, he saw the Hu brothers.

"Master Liu," said the elder. "The villagers wanted to show once again their appreciation for what you did. Some of them want you to stay permanently and be part of this village. Is there any way or anything we can do to convince you to stay? We would be willing to pay you appropriately, and provide you with a place to live along with whatever food you require."

"Once again, I appreciate the offer, but for the time being it is out of the question. We need to discuss my situation as soon as possible."

"Master, I have briefly discussed your problem with the Hu brothers. They are willing to listen to what you have to say. May I also be part of the conversation?"

"Of course, please come in. I have some water boiling for tea."

"Master, none of us have had breakfast. I have taken the liberty of asking one of the women of the village to prepare something for the five of us. She and her daughter made that fine meal for you and Pei Ke when you were here before. She will also have one of the men bring some more chairs so that we all can sit and relax as we eat and talk."

Liu remembered the woman and her daughter. He smiled to himself as he remembered how hard she had worked to get Pei Ke to pay attention to her daughter. It was no more than thirty seconds after Liu shut the door, than there was a knock and she stood with her daughter carrying trays of food, more food than five men could possibly eat.

"Master Liu, we have brought some breakfast for you, Pei Ke, and the rest of the men. We hope that Pei Ke likes it. My daughter cooked something special for him."

She looked around to see if Pei Ke was there.

"It is very kind of you to cook this," said Liu. "Unfortunately, Pei Ke is not with me this trip. I will see him in a couple of days and I will mention that you and your daughter cooked something special for him. I am sure that he would have liked to be here to partake of it, but I have him doing a special errand for me. Maybe he will come back in the near future."

The woman looked disappointed and not surprisingly, the daughter looked disappointed as well. They brought the food in and placed it on the table. Two men behind them brought in some chairs and then they all left, leaving Liu, the village elder, and the Hu brothers.

"Please sit down," said Liu. "Thank you for coming and I want to thank the village elder for bringing you here. I again want to thank you three for helping us when we were last here, and I was impressed by your martial arts abilities and willingness to help others."

"We martial artists are all part of a brotherhood. Regardless of the style and lineage, we have respect for each other's abilities. The elder has explained that you wanted to talk with us. He has given us a very brief explanation, but we would like to hear it from you with more details. We do not want any surprises. As you know, the villagers have hired us to protect them. We are aware that they offered the position to you first and you declined for various reasons."

"First of all, I am not here to take over your position. I am here only to enlist your professional help and of course I am willing to pay you for your services."

Liu sipped his tea and the others followed suit. As the others were eating, Liu began to share with them his background. He explained what had happened over the years to bring these past events to a current crisis. Liu explained everything that was material to the situation, including his suspicion that the Abbot of the temple was somehow involved, either in a direct or indirect way.

After two hours of discussion with everyone expressing their particular viewpoint, a course of action was agreed upon.

CHAPTER 45

Pei Ke covered the remaining distance to Wei Ken De's in record time and without further incident. He went to the front gate and rang the bell. After a moment, the door opened and he saw the same person he had seen when he and Liu first went to visit Wei Ken De.

There was instant recognition on the man's part as he opened the door and waved him in.

"I do not see Master Liu. Is he with you?"

"No," said Pei Ke.

"Will he be coming later?"

"Maybe. Is Wei Ken De here?"

"No, he is out for the day. However, Mei Li is here. Would you like to see her?"

"Yes, please."

The man escorted Pei Ke through the courtyard and into the main house and the sitting room.

"Mei Li is working outside right now, I will get her. She will be here in a few minutes. Please have a seat."

Pei Ke remembered the room from the first time he'd met Wei Ken De. He sat down in the same chair he'd sat in before. He looked around, than changed to the chair Liu sat in weeks earlier. As he sat in the chair, he felt more at ease. He was no longer a fledging student, but one accepted into the tradition of the Liu family. He wanted Mei Li to realize this from the start.

He was happy Wei Ken De was gone. He wanted to talk with Mei Li privately. He considered how he was going to start the conversation. As he was formulating the words in his head, he realized he'd been waiting for more than a few minutes. It had been at least twenty minutes since the servant had left. Maybe she was some distance away from the house. What could possibly be taking her so long?

Just as he was about to get up, he heard someone running down the hallway. The running stopped just outside the door to the sitting room. Pei Ke expected the door to open, but nothing happened. Five seconds went by, then ten seconds went by, and then the door slowly opened.

Mei Li walked into the room wearing a beautiful silk outfit. Her hair was fashioned in an exquisite bow with a needle in the center to keep it in place. Pei Ke could not remember her looking so beautiful and he stood up as Mei Li bowed. He returned the bow. The two of them just looked at each other; neither one quite knew what to say. Mei Li broke the awkward silence.

"Pei Ke, you have returned. We did not expect you or Master Liu to return for some time. Is he here as well?"

Pei Ke just stood there, not knowing what to say. He hadn't been prepared for her stunning beauty. Again, Mei Li broke the silence.

"Where is Master Liu?"

"He didn't come. I came by myself."

Mei Li's heart skipped a beat. She wondered if he had come for her. She looked into his eyes, and smiling indicated for him to sit down. As she sat in the chair next to him, the door opened and the servant entered the room. Pei Ke was surprised he did not knock, and then realized the servant was doing his duty to protect Mei Li.

"It is alright," said Mei Li. "Pei Ke is here to share information. Would you be so kind as to tell the other servants to bring us some of our best tea?"

The servant looked directly at Pei Ke. The nonverbal communication between the two of them was very clear. The servant bowed and closed the door. Pei Ke was impressed with how dedicated and protective the servant was towards Mei Li.

"Mei Li, you look beautiful."

She blushed and cast her eyes downward as her heart raced even faster than it did before. She had waited for Pei Ke and he had returned. He had all the attributes a woman would want in a man. She would do everything in her power to prevent him from getting away again.

"I am sure you did not come this far just to tell me that."

She waited for a reply ever woman wants to hear. Her heart was full of joy and happiness. If what she expected was true, she was going to be the happiest woman in the world.

"You are beautiful, but I'm afraid you're correct. I've come on a very urgent matter, and I need to talk with you and your father as soon as possible."

Her heart sank a little.

"Is Master Liu alright?"

"Yes and no. I really don't know. I haven't seen him for two days. He sent me here, while he went east to visit some villagers. It's a long story, though, and I'd rather not tell it twice. Where is your father?"

"He is out. I expect him back in an hour, two hours at the most. I know you want to talk to him, but is there anything you can share with me?"

Pei Ke started to share what had happened from the time they had left Wei Ken De's place. The servant knocked and then walked in with the tea. They both watched in silence as the servant put the teapot and three cups on the table and then left.

When the door closed, it was immediately reopened and Wei Ken De entered the room.

"Father, you are home early. Look, Pei Ke is here."

Without even acknowledging Mei Li, he walked over to Pei Ke. Pei Ke stood up and bowed to his martial art brother. Wei Ken De bowed slightly and motioned for him to sit. Wei Ken De noticed Pei Ke was sitting in the chair Liu had sat in before.

"Where is Master Liu?"

"It is a long story, and I need to explain to both of you why I am here."

"Is he alright?" asked Wei Ken De.

"Yes, he is alright. Or he was when I last saw him two days ago."

Pei Ke opened his shirt, took out the paper Liu had given him in the restaurant, and carefully handed it to Wei Ken De.

"Teacher told me to come here and give you this letter. I am also to bring you up to date in detail on where we have been and what has taken place since we left here."

Wei Ken De nodded, then read and reread the letter and then gave it to Mei Li.

"Have you read this letter?"

"No. Teacher folded it and told me to safeguard it and to give it to you. He didn't tell me to read it."

"So you have no idea what it says. Is that correct?"

"No, though I'd guess it involves teacher asking you for some help in dealing with the attacks on his family and himself."

"No, it doesn't say that at all."

Wei Ken De watched Mei Li, waiting for her to finish reading the letter. When she finished she glanced at Pei Ke and then looked at her father and smiled. Then both looked at Pei Ke and smiled.

"The letter says that you…"

CHAPTER 46

Chen and his men arrived at the Liu compound and scouted the area for any activity. There was no outward sign that anyone was there, so he became concerned for the two men he'd dispatched ahead of the group. They should have been there to meet him and he had a sinking feeling that Liu had outmaneuvered him again.

He sent two of his men over the wall and minutes later, the gate opened and they emerged.

"No one's here," said one of the men. "There are some hoof prints, but the place is deserted."

"I was told Liu and his student would be here," said Chen. "Obviously, the information was wrong. Well, we're here now, and we're going to stay for a couple of days until we find out where he is hiding.

"Even though Liu is not here now, I don't want him to surprise us at night. Rotate three-hour shifts of two men each. From past experience, Liu will try to sneak up on us when we least expect it. So keep the gate locked at all times."

CHAPTER 47

Liu and two of the Hu brothers said goodbye to the villagers and rode west away from the village. One of the brothers volunteered to stay behind to protect the villagers. This was not what Liu wanted, but two additional men were better than no men at all. He wished he could get men from his own village, but they were farmers, and not fighters. They would probably be killed instantly. He could not ask them, and the local constable was totally useless.

The three rode quickly toward Liu's ancestral village. They pushed the horses hard, resting only when it was absolutely necessary. After a quick journey, Liu and his two companions rode into the village in the early evening. Liu nodded to some of the villagers as they made their way home for the evening. As they rode up to the temple, Liu looked around but could see nothing out of the ordinary. He suggested that the two brothers stay on their horses. He would only be a minute.

He walked into the temple and went straight to the Abbot's office. He was initially greeted by Abbot's assistant, who appeared surprised to see him. The assistant was about to say something when the door opened and the Abbot emerged.

"Master Liu, it is you again."

"Are you surprised to see me?" asked Liu.

"No, we are always happy to see you. Come into my office and sit. Do you want some tea?"

"No, tea is not necessary. I have been away for a few days and wanted to find out if anyone had seen or heard of any strangers coming into the village or the surrounding area?"

"I have not heard of any strangers. Are you expecting anyone in particular?"

"Well, those who killed Wu may still be around. If so, I would like to know where they are. I feel certain whoever killed Wu also killed the servant boy and possibly had something to do with the death of my family."

The Abbot did not answer; he simply shrugged his shoulders. Liu looked into his eyes and was certain the man was either withholding information or was lying.

"I need to visit Wu's place and see if there are any more clues. Have you or anyone else been to his place since the massacre?"

"To my knowledge, no one from the temple has been there since the attack. We are shocked by the chain of events that have taken place, and hopefully, those who have committed these heinous crimes can be brought to justice. Do you have any idea who they might be?"

"No, but there may be some clues at Wu's place. Are there any other places where you think I might find out more information or discover some clues?"

"No. Where are you going now?"

"I will be going to Wu's and will stay there tonight and tomorrow night. I will be back in the village in two days, and we can discuss the amulets at that time. I have decided to change the distribution of what was left by my father."

The Abbot's eyes widened.

"Master Liu, I was given very specific instructions concerning what should be done with the estate once the four coins are presented to me."

"What instructions were you given if the coins were missing and not held by their rightful owners?"

Liu did not wait for an answer. He looked into the Abbot's eyes and bowed slightly, then left. The Abbot was deep in thought as Liu walked out the door. Minutes later the Abbot walked out the door and went to the street in front of the temple. He saw Liu and two men riding south away from the temple on the road to Wu's place. He did not know the men and it did not register with him whether or not he should find out who they were.

The Abbot quickly went back to his office and scribbled a note on some rice paper. He folded the paper, put a drop of candle wax on it to seal it from prying eyes, and went in search of one of the monks. When he found the monk, he gave him the note with explicit instructions to whom to give it. The monk understood the importance of finding the right person and left immediately.

CHAPTER 48

Liu and his companions rode south and took the cut-off to Wu's estate. The possibility of finding any clues was remote, but it was a good place for them to start. Chen would have no legitimate reason to stay there, so he would likely have moved on. He certainly would not want to implicate himself. If he thought Liu was there, however, he'd certainly return and attack.

Liu and his two companions arrived at Wu's place and found it was just as he had left it. No one had come to clean up the mess created by the attackers and the dried blood remained where it had been spilled.

"Someone really made a mess of this place," said one of the Hu brothers. "Whoever did this was looking for something. It doesn't look like they just wanted to destroy things. There was a purpose to what they did."

"Yes," said Liu. "They were looking for anything of value that they could take with them. Other than nice furniture and some paintings and vases, there was nothing of value to the attackers. Of course, these things are of value to someone who wants to live here."

"How long are we going to wait?" asked one of the brothers. "Are we planning to wait for them to attack us, or are we going to attack them first?"

"I do not want to attack them first, unless I have a definite advantage. It might be best if they initiate the attack so we can be certain that it is them who committed the crime. If we attack them, any survivors could say that we were the aggressors and that can't happen. This must be the final altercation.

"We also need to wait for Wei Ken De and Pei Ke to arrive, which should be today or tomorrow. In the meantime, I would like to clean up this place and put the furniture and cabinets back where they belong. It shouldn't take too much time if we work together."

For the remainder of the day Liu and his companions straightened up Wu's place putting the house back in order the best they could and taking out things that were broken beyond repair. When they were finished, Liu walked around the house and looked at what remained of a once beautiful home.

At night, they took turns on guard while the other two slept, though Liu was sure Chen would not attack before the following day.

CHAPTER 49

C hen wondered what to do next. He had several alternatives. He could wait at the Liu compound for Liu to come to him, or he could hunt Liu and attack him wherever he found him.

According to the monk who brought the note, Liu was at Wu's place, but that made no sense. Why would Liu go to Wu's when this was his ancestral home. Maybe the note was wrong. Maybe it was a trick by the Abbot to get him off guard and allow Liu to attack him. He discounted that thought as the Abbot was too deeply involved and had no choice but to continue to supply him information.

He was sure the Abbot knew where the Liu family hid the treasure. There was no other reason for Liu Bin to be so friendly with him. Either way, Chen was sure the Abbot was waiting to see which way the wind was blowing before fully committing to one side or another.

If Liu were dead, then the Abbot would have no choice but to deal with Chen. Chen felt sure the two amulets now in his possession were a key to the Liu fortune. Why else would the servant boy and the girl be carrying them around their necks?

Chen took the two amulets from around his neck. Looking at them, he guessed there were two more to make the amulet one whole piece. He tried to put the two pieces he had together, but they would not match. He surmised that he only had the pieces opposite each other. He did not have the two pieces that were next to each other.

He was almost sure the Abbot had one of the amulets; otherwise, Liu would not be so friendly with the Abbot. The two pieces he did not have were critical for him to solve the puzzle. Even if he did have the other two amulets, what did it mean? Was it a clue to a location or was it information on the lands? Or, maybe it was information on the lineage of the Liu family. Whatever it was, the Abbot had something to do with it.

Chen also thought about why the Abbot was willing to help him. If the Abbot knew the location of the treasure, why didn't he just take it and leave? He immediately knew the answer. He was afraid of Liu. Once Liu was out of the way, the Abbot could then do whatever he needed to do to claim a portion of the fortune. But, why did the Abbot want the Liu fortune and lands? As a Buddhist monk, he was supposed to eschew worldly needs. All needs were to be provided for him. There must be a flaw in the Abbot's personality. Maybe he had seen the lifestyle of Liu and his family and wanted some of it for himself.

It did not matter what the situation was, the Abbot was not going to be part of the distribution of the land and fortune. Everything was going to be his, just the way his father had wanted it. He would deal with the Abbot at the appropriate time. First things first, he needed to get rid of Liu.

Chen stood up from his chair and went outside. As he walked around the Liu compound, he was satisfied that the rotating guards would be able to sound the alarm in plenty of time if attacked.

CHAPTER 50

Pei Ke explained to Wei Ken De everything that had transpired since he and Liu had departed weeks earlier. He told them about the trip to Beijing and the various attacks along the way. He explained the meeting with Sun and the revelation that Hua Yee was in danger. With tears in his eyes, he explained her untimely death, and the death of the servant boy.

Now Liu was in danger and it was more than he could handle by himself. Of course, Wei Ken De was ready to help, and even Wei Ken De's servant was willing to help. Mei Li even volunteered to come, but her father ruled against it. He needed someone to take care of the business and run the estate while he was gone. The servant and Mei Li were to stay behind and take care of business.

The relationship between Wei Ken De and Pei Ke changed on this visit. The letter Pei Ke carried to Wei Ken De described how Pei Ke was now accepted fully into the Liu family as an inner door student, and was entitled to the benefits of learning not only from Liu, but also from his most senior students. Wei Ken De conveyed this information to Pei Ke who was overwhelmed that Liu would send such a note to his senior student. Pei Ke now held the same status as Wei Ken De, but on a junior level.

That night it was agreed Pei Ke and Wei Ken De would leave as soon as there was light. Pei Ke was given a room for the night. Late in the evening, Mei Li and her father sat by themselves in the main sitting room.

"Father, I would like to go with you two in the morning. You have taught me well and I can handle myself."

"Yes, my daughter, you have learned well and I have no doubt that you could handle yourself, but I need someone to be here to look after the business and take care of the house. When your mother was alive, and we knew we could have no more children, we decided to entrust you with everything you needed to know to carry on the traditions of this family. That included running the business and the house.

"I have been here to guide you and now it is your turn to step forward and to take charge while I am absent. It is not a matter of your martial arts abilities, but of the priorities of the moment. Do you understand?"

"Yes, father. When you put it that way, I do understand. I will do my best." She looked disappointed but was resigned to the circumstances.

"If I had any doubts about your capabilities, I would not have you assume this responsibility."

"Father, I will stay and take care of the business and the household duties."

"Good."

She looked thoughtfully into the fireplace and for a brief moment watched the flames dance.

"Father I want to talk with you for a few minutes before we go to bed."

"What is it?"

"I am now of age, and my girlfriends are either married or they are promised to someone. I was wondering if you had considered my future?"

"The matchmaker has contacted me about some suitable young men in the area. I know who they are and, while I am not overly impressed with them, they do come from good families and each would be a match which would solidify the families together."

"Father, do I know any of these young men?"

"One is the son of a millwright. His father has a very good business."

Mei Li gasped slightly.

"Father, if it is who I think it is; that boy is an idiot. I've talked with him and he has nothing intelligent to say. You can't possibly be serious."

Wei Ken De smiled slightly.

"Well, I haven't met him yet."

"What about the other one?"

"His father owns a farm out in the countryside."

"Father, can you see me working on a farm isolated in the countryside."

"When your mother and I decided to educate you and to help make you self-sufficient, we were warned that someday you would want to be in charge of your own destiny. In some respects, this goes counter to all our traditions both in our culture and in our family. On the other hand, I am all for someone who wants to be in charge of their own destiny. I have to balance our customs with your independence. Whatever decision I make will be for your own good and the good of this family."

"Father, I want…" She saw his arched eyebrow and started again. Excuse me, I would like for you to consider Pei Ke as a suitable husband for me. I will not find anyone more loyal and considerate than him. I realize he does not have the family status we have, but his other qualities are far superior to the two who you mentioned.

"He is already linked to us through Liu Bin. He highly respects you, and most of all he would do honor to you, to Liu, and to our own family."

"Have you mentioned anything to him about this?"

"Father! Of course not. I would be too embarrassed to mention this subject. It is not proper for a young lady to do so; however, it is proper for you as my father to initiate this discussion. Since he has no family, however, it seems appropriate for you to also mention it to Liu Bin. Don't you think that would be a good idea? In this way you could take the lead and make all the decisions."

Wei Ken De looked at his daughter and smiled to himself how she had twisted the situation around so that it appeared he was making the decision. She will do well in business as a negotiator, he thought.

"It is getting late and Pei Ke and I have to leave at first light. Get some sleep daughter. This topic and a resolution to it is not that important right now. Let me ask you a question. Is there a reason that I need to make a decision at this moment?"

"No father, there is time enough for us to further address this subject at a later time. It's just that my girlfriends are all getting married and at age nineteen, I am feeling old and left out. Some of them have already started a family, and I also would like to have a family."

"Go to bed now," said Wei Ken De. "I promise to think seriously about it; however, whatever decision I make I expect you to follow my wishes."

"Yes, father."

Mei Li went to her bedroom, changed into her nightclothes, and laid in bed thinking about her conversation with her father. After an hour of random thoughts, she rose and put on a covering and walked down the hallway to Pei Ke's room. She carefully opened the door and looked in. She could hear the softness of his breathing. She tiptoed into the room, but left the door slightly ajar to let in light. She walked to his bed, looked at him, wondering what it would be like to be married to him. Yes, there were families who had a rich tradition and he had none. There were men who could always provide her with luxury, and at the moment, he had nothing. There were also men more handsome than he, but they were usually egotistical.

She walked around to the other side of the bed and gently touched the extra pillow. She stared at the bed and then at Pei Ke, and then back at the bed. She felt an ache in her body as she retraced her steps back to her room. She laid in bed thinking about the conversation she had with her father. He was right about the way she had been brought up. Yes, she had her girlfriends and they would get together and talk as young girls would talk, but she always felt that they were too immature.

As she grew older, the gulf between the maturity levels only increased. She was thankful she was brought up the way she was and not like the other girls. None of her girlfriends knew martial arts. None of her girlfriends knew how to run a business. None of her girlfriends knew how to ride a horse. She wondered if she was acting too much like a boy or a man and not enough like a girl or a woman. Pei Ke, or whomever her husband was going to be, needed to know she had not been brought up like most other girls and she was happy with what she had become. She was thankful to her father for her upbringing.

She was positive she was making the right selection and knew in her heart Pei Ke would make the perfect husband. If only she could get her father to see it the way she saw it. She needed to talk with Liu Bin. Her father would listen to him. She just needed the right moment.

The following day, Wei Ken De and Pei Ke traveled north as fast as they could. Pei Ke had a fresh horse from Wei Ken De's stable. If they pushed the horses hard, they could make it to Wu's place the next day.

CHAPTER 51

Wei Ken De and Pei Ke had been riding most of the second day when they trotted up to the front of the Wu compound. From the outside, it looked totally deserted and the gate was closed.

"Are you sure this is where we're supposed to meet Teacher?" Wei Ken De said as they approached.

"Yes," said Pei Ke. "Look, there's one of the Hu brother's by the gate."

Pei Ke nodded to the man and he let them pass into the compound. As soon as they were inside, he shut and bolted the gate. They rode up to the main house and went inside. Liu and one of the other brothers were there. The other brother walked in shortly thereafter, and Liu made the introductions.

"Master, it is good to see you again," said Wei Ken De as he bowed to his teacher. "You have been through a lot and hopefully I can help you."

"Come in Wei Ken De," said Liu. "It is true a lot has happened since we were last together, and I assume Pei Ke has shared with you all the relevant details. I need to put an end to all of this mess as soon as possible. We can talk later, but right now let's get acquainted."

Liu looked at each of them, aware that they were sizing each other up. He understood and wanted to make it easier for each of them since they were all accomplished martial artists.

"I want to thank each of you for coming here. Although this is my fight and not yours, I appreciate your willingness to help. Each of you knows the relevant facts in this situation, but let me review. Basically, Chen claims ownership of my ancestral land and any fortune associated with it. He has no legitimate claim to this land, and this fact has been substantiated by the Emperor's official office. Chen has amassed a group of men, who are not martial artists like us, but are proficient fighters nonetheless. His plan is to kill me and then claim the land.

"I would prefer not to initiate an attack against him and his men, but would rather have them attack us first. That way we are justified in the actions we will have to take. As of now, I suspect that they have taken over my home and lands.

I do not want any of you to feel guilt or remorse in what is going to happen. Hopefully, none of us will be hurt and we can stop Chen in his tracks."

"What is our course of action?" asked one of the Hu brothers.

"As I just indicated I think Chen and his men are north of here at my ancestral home. He is likely trying to decide what to do. It would be ideal for him to leave my home so we can enter and secure the compound. It will be easier for us to fight from an area I am familiar with rather than an area not known to any of us. He probably thinks that if he occupies the place long enough it will be his. Or, if I return to it he can kill me and have no one to contest his ownership.

"For now, we are going to rest, and we will all take our turn at guard duty tonight. It would be good for all of you to become better acquainted. We are going to be relying on each other during the next few days, and I want to make sure that we are all comfortable with each other."

"Master," said Pei Ke. "You are probably correct in your estimation of where Chen is going. When I was heading south from the village to go to Wei Ken De's place I was attacked by two of Chen's men. They are now lying dead and I hid their bodies in the forest. About an hour after the encounter while I was covering up their bodies a group of about ten men rode past. I was too far into the forest to get a look at them but I assume it was Chen and his men."

"How do you know the two men were Chen's men?" asked Liu.

"They seemed to know who I was when they attacked me."

Liu looked at Wei Ken De and then the Hu brothers. Liu smiled and nodded.

"You did well," said Liu.

Pei Ke looked at Wei Ken De but Wei Ken De remained expressionless.

For the next couple of hours, the newly formed group shared information about themselves with emphasis on their martial arts training and experience. It was evident to each of them, that everyone was an accomplished martial artist except for Pei Ke. Even though he had taken care of two of Chen's men, he was not an accomplished martial artist and possibly the weak link in the group.

That night the men discussed strategy and a course of action for the next day. They agreed they would stay the night and have Pei Ke go into town the following morning and get supplies.

Pei Ke took the first watch for two hours and then had one of the Hu brothers take over the next shift. As the others slept, Liu and We Ken De talked. It was an opportunity for Liu to share more information with Wei Ken De about what had transpired. He trusted his senior student and felt the bond they had developed over the years was more than a teacher student relationship.

It was also time for Wei Ken De to understand the depth of Liu's anguish. Pei Ke had given details, but he could not impart to Wei Ken De the emotional heartache Liu had endured at the hands of Chen and his men. No one could understand unless they were able to sense the emotions behind the words, and this is what he wanted to convey to Wei Ken De.

As it got late, Liu suggested they continue their conversation at another time. It was important for both of them to get as much rest as possible. Liu went to one of the bedrooms. No sooner was his head on the pillow than he felt a change in the Universal Energy. He was sure it was Chen plotting his evil ways.

———————————

Chen went to sleep that night satisfied with what had happened so far. He was in possession of the land and the compound. The magistrate would do nothing to evict him. He had shown the magistrate the document signed by a well-known warlord, giving his father the lands and the compound. There was nothing the magistrate was going to do to challenge that information and he was sure the magistrate had mentioned it to some of the other villagers. Those villagers were not going to throw him off the property on their own.

The Abbot was on his side, and was giving him information on a regular basis. The Abbot was a fool. Chen knew the Abbot was playing both sides, waiting for a clear winner. He would take care of the Abbot later. Right now, he needed him.

His primary focus was to eliminate Liu and his student, once and for all. What could two men do against the men he now had? Even if Liu was a master of martial arts, he could not prevail against all his men. He did not stand a chance. All they needed to do was to keep vigilant and stay where they were for as long as possible. Liu must know by now that he is going to lose. He must be afraid. In the morning, he would send one of his men into town to get some supplies. This was going to be a long ordeal. His father would be proud of him for staying the course and retrieving what rightfully belonged in the Chen family. As he stretched out in bed, he went over in his head various scenarios that could take place in the coming days. Satisfied he had thought of everything, he thought of his wife and son who were waiting for him. He smiled to himself as he fell asleep.

CHAPTER 52

The next morning Pei Ke woke up just as it was becoming daylight. He had not slept well. He'd dreamt of Hua Yee and how she must have suffered before she died on the mountain. She was so close to her home. The more he thought about what happened to her the angrier he became.

Pei Ke walked into the sitting room to find Liu and Wei Ken De already up and in a conversation.

"Where are the Hu brothers?" asked Pei Ke.

"One is still asleep and the other is on guard duty," said Liu. "Did you sleep well?"

"No. There were too many things going through my head. Many things that needed to be resolved won't get resolved for a while."

"Pei Ke, as we discussed last night, I want you to go to the village. When you get there, go to the market, and get some rice and some other supplies. I want you to spend a little time in the village so the villagers will know you are there. Get enough supplies to last us a couple of days. Take an extra horse with you."

"Here are some coins," said Wei Ken De. "This should be enough to cover the cost of what you buy."

"I want you to go now, and remember to spend enough time in the village so they know you are there, but do not make it too obvious. Is that clear?" asked Liu.

"Yes, Master," said Pei Ke.

Pei Ke left the room and went to the stable. After getting the horses ready, he rode out of the stable. Liu and Wei Ken De were watching as Pei Ke rode away from Wu's estate. Little did Liu and Wei Ken De know that Pei Ke would again be tested to his fullest.

"Master, he is very loyal to you," said Wei Ken De. "He is a good student. Your note said that you had accepted him as an inner door student. It is none of my business, but you accepted him quite early. Is he that good in martial arts?"

"He learns fast and he remembers. He reminds me of you when you first came to me to study. He will do well. That brings up a point I want to discuss with you. I think he needs to study from you for a while. Even though you follow my teachings, you have your own viewpoint on what you have learned. That is where the wisdom of the teacher and student come into play. The teacher can only show the way. It is up to the student to grasp the material. Then, the student can tailor the material to suit his or her needs. I am sure you teach your daughter a little differently than I taught you. Your insight into the arts helps you to adapt the material to her needs. Pei Ke needs to see the material from another viewpoint for him to realize his potential."

"So you think he can become an accomplished martial artist?" asked Wei Ken De.

"Yes, it is possible with the right guidance. I think you are the person to do it. I have taught him much of what he needs to know over a very short period of time. He needs to have that material reinforced a few times and presented in a different way. He needs to be challenged in actual fighting to solidify what he knows. He needs to know he can actually use it when called upon. He is still a little hesitant in that respect, but he is getting better."

"How will he do when we meet up with Chen?"

"According to him he was able to handle the two men who attacked him. Of course, we don't know the circumstances, but I suspect that these two men were not very good and Pei Ke was lucky. If his opponent is simply average, then he might be able to handle himself. If his opponent is an accomplished martial artist, he will have a difficult time."

"Master, how old is Pei Ke?" asked Wei Ken De.

Liu chuckled.

"It is strange you ask. I do not remember asking him, and if I did ask him, I do not remember what he said. My guess is that he is in his early to middle twenties. Why do you ask?"

"Mei Li has mentioned that many of her girlfriends are married or have been promised to another family. I have not been diligent in finding her a suitable husband. She has reminded me of my responsibilities in this matter. She doesn't think much of the men in our area. Those who are available from good families are either, according to her, 'idiots' or uninteresting. I need for her to marry into a good family."

"As you know with the death of Hua Yee and the small children I do not have any recognized heirs to the Liu estate."

"Master, at one time you mentioned your parents also had a daughter. Where is she?"

"She married and went with her husband, but sadly, she died not too long ago and did not leave any children. So, there really is no one left. I have accepted Pei Ke into my family just as I have accepted you and a few others into my family to carry on the traditions of my martial arts and my teachings. You and the others are family to me. Now this is true of Pei Ke as well. He is now family to me. Would someone in my family, whom I trust and deem worthy, be an acceptable husband for your daughter?"

CHAPTER 53

As Pei Ke rode north from the Wu compound toward the village, one of Chen's men rode south from Liu's ancestral home toward the village. They had never met nor had they even seen the other. They had both departed early in the morning with very specific instructions.

Pei Ke was to get supplies and make his presence known to the villagers. Hopefully, the word would get back to Chen that Liu was staying away from his ancestral home. Chen's man was also to get supplies, and visit with the Abbot to get an update about Liu's whereabouts.

Pei Ke arrived first and went to the restaurant he and Liu had gone to before. When he walked into the restaurant, he could see only a few morning patrons. He nodded to the owner, who recognized him, and headed to the far wall, nodding to the various patrons seated for breakfast. He sat down at a table away from the others with his back to the wall and watched as the others ate their food. Minutes later, the owner came over.

"You are Pei Ke, right?" said the restaurant owner.

"Yes, I'm glad you remembered."

"You were with Liu Bin. We have known each other for a long time. Will he be joining you for breakfast?"

"No, I came to the village this morning to pick up some supplies. Teacher gave me a long list of things to get. However, I could not resist coming here since I haven't eaten this morning. I remembered how good the food was last time and I'm sure the food is going to be just as good this time. Right?"

"Of course, the food is always good. What would you like?"

"I would like hot tea, porridge, and dumplings."

Pei Ke motioned for the restaurant owner to sit down. In a lowered voice, he asked the restaurant owner.

"Is there anything you think is important for Liu to know? When I finish eating I will be going to get supplies and then leaving."

The man shook his head, but then he said.

"Nothing is new here. I have not heard anyone discussing anything of importance. The only strange thing is that the Abbot is on the street more than usual. It is customary for him to be in the temple attending to his duties there, but I've seen him on the street at some odd times. The reason I know is that I go to the market during the slack hours and get whatever produce I need."

"I thought the market was only open during the early morning?"

"Yes, basically, that is true. Most of the vendors close early because they have already sold their produce for the day. However, there are a couple of shop keepers who stay open all day. They sell not only produce but also some dry goods. I get the few produce items that I need at these shops."

"When does the produce market close?"

"It will close in maybe another hour. You have time to relax and enjoy your meal. I will go and get it ready for you."

"Thank you."

Pei Ke ate his breakfast. When he finished, most of the patrons had gone. He paid for his meal, walked out the door, and headed for the temple to get the horses. When he left the horses in front of the temple, he knew they would be safe, for very few people would steal horses that were next to a place of worship.

He pulled on the reins and walked his horses down the street to the market to get the needed supplies. While he was at the market, he went out of his way to talk with the locals. He had never had the opportunity to converse with them and he found them very friendly and outgoing.

"This village would be a nice place to live," thought Pei Ke, as he put the supplies on the horse.

CHAPTER 54

The Abbot looked up from his desk as one of the monks walked into his office.

"There's a man here to see you," said the monk.

"Who is he?" replied the Abbot.

"I asked, but he just said that he was a friend of a friend and he wanted to see you. He said it was important."

The Abbot thought for a moment and then replied.

"Send him in."

The man walked in and stood in front of the Abbot's desk. He did not bow or show any respect.

"Chen suggested I come here and see if you have any more information for him."

"I told him that he and his men should not come here. I can't be seen with him or any of his men. There is nothing for me to tell you that he does not already know. Now go, and leave me alone, and do not come back here."

"I've come for supplies and Chen said you would be able to give me some money."

"We have no money except what is given to us by those who pray here. Most of what we have given to us is food as a sacrifice by the villagers. Why does he think we have any money?"

"I do not know. He just said you'd give it to me."

There was a knock on the door and one of the monks entered without being invited to do so. This surprised the Abbot who looked upset at the intrusion.

"I am sorry to disturb you," said the monk. "It is important."

"Yes," said the Abbot.

The monk walked in, and went over to the Abbot's side so he could whisper in the Abbot's ear.

"Pei Ke is in the village getting supplies and he is by himself," said the monk.

"Where is he now?" The Abbot made no attempt to whisper.

"He is at the market," whispered the monk. "He has already bought supplies and is getting ready to leave."

"Where is he going?"

The man just stood there trying to absorb and understand the conversation.

"We do not know."

The Abbot thought for a few minutes. He looked at the man Chen had sent and then at the monk. He did not want to involve the monk, but if he could eliminate Pei Ke, then it would be easier for him to accomplish his objective. Chen and his men could easily handle just one man even if it was Liu. No man could fight numerous men at one time. It was impossible. Once Liu was killed, he would then implicate Chen in the killings. With Chen gone there would be no one else in the way of his claiming the Liu ancestral land for the temple. He knew where the treasure was hidden, and he was sure there was documentation with the treasure, outlining the distribution of the wealth. He just needed the other two amulets to make sure there was no way anything could be traced to him or the temple.

He turned to the monk.

"Find Pei Ke and tell him I want to see him by the stream where we draw the water. Tell him I am there now and that I've discovered something that will help Liu solve the death of the servant boy."

The monk left the room and the Chen's man watched him leave. Excitedly, he bent forward and in a subdued voice he asked.

"Is this the person who is traveling with Liu?"

"Yes, it is. His name is Pei Ke and he is one of the individuals your boss is trying to eliminate. Chen would be really pleased with you if you could help solve one of his problems."

The Abbot smiled and nodded to the man. The man grinned.

"Do you know where the stream is located?" asked the Abbot.

"No, but I can find it. Just point me in the right direction."

The Abbot pointed to the rear of the temple.

"There is a path at the back of the temple. It goes through a wooded area which is quite secluded. We are the only ones who use it. You do not need to come back here and please do not leave anything at the stream. We like to keep the area clean. When you leave do not come back through the village. Cross over the stream and circle around the west side of the village. There may be a couple of horses with some supplies you may want to add to your collection.

The Abbot looked down at the pieces of rice paper that were on his desk. Inwardly he smiled to himself. Things were starting to fall into place. The man turned and departed. Neither one of them made eye contact with the other.

As the man departed from the temple, the Abbot knew that his fate was sealed one way or the other. He was sure Liu suspected something, but there was no way he could prove it. If this coming altercation worked as he hoped it would, then everything would be fine. If it did not work out the way he hoped, then everything would remain just as before. He had always wanted to live in the countryside, especially the valley where the Liu family had resided. He wondered if they had really acquired it legally.

Chapter 55

Walking behind the temple, Pei Ke easily found the path leading down to the stream. He had never been here before, in fact, he hadn't even known that it even existed. Even though the path was narrow, it was wide enough for him to guide his horse and the extra horse carrying the supplies.

He thought it interesting and somewhat disconcerting that the Abbot wanted to show him some clues concerning the death of Chang Song. He didn't trust the Abbot and was sure that the Abbot was somehow involved in the terrible events that had taken place. Chang Song's death had been a terrible tragedy. If there were really some clues, Liu Bin would be interested in anything that would shed light on who had killed the boy. Maybe he was wrong about the Abbot.

Walking down the sloping path he thought of Hua Yee. It was beyond his imagination how his teacher could process all the grief and still be calm. His attention turned to the mixture of pine and regular leafy trees. The branches of the leaf bearing trees still had no leaves on them. It was too early for the buds to come out. However, the day was not as cold as previous days had been. If the temperature improved over the next three weeks, there would definitely be a sign of spring. Hua Yee would probably have liked this scene.

Pei Ke noticed a slight drop in temperature as the path continued sloping downward. He then felt a chill go through his body, unlike anything he'd experienced before. It was intense, a foreboding chill that something sinister was about to happen.

He had felt this before with Liu, but this time he was alone and it really was intense. He shook his head to disperse the feeling and thoughts. Just then, he heard the rustle of leaves and a movement to his right. He turned in time to see a man rushing toward him with a broadsword raised ready to attack. As the man approached, all sense of time briefly froze for Pei Ke.

He saw the broadsword arcing downward toward his head. He stepped to the left to get out of the centerline of the attack. He wasn't fast enough and the tip of the blade sliced through his shirt making a shallow cut on his shoulder. Pei Ke immediately felt the pain. Blood dripped from his shoulder and ran down his sleeve. Everything sped up at that moment. Pei Ke's left hand came around as he turned slightly to face his assailant. He grabbed the man's right wrist with his left hand. With his right, he grabbed underneath the man's wrist and applied a Chin Na technique to the wrist. The man screamed and immediately dropped the broadsword. Pei Ke struck toward the man's face with his right fist, but the man ducked and the punch went wide of its mark.

The assailant yanked his right wrist free of Pei Ke's grab and leaned down to pick up the broadsword, but Pei Ke stepped on the blade with his left foot, then with his right heel, kicked the man in the jaw as hard as he could.

The man fell to the ground and Pei Ke picked up the broadsword with his left hand, than moved in. He swung the broadsword at the man's head, but the assailant rolled to one side and the blade struck the ground. He continued rolling, than stood before Pei Ke could strike again.

Pei Ke realized that he didn't know the first thing about how to use a broadsword, but he was thankful he'd disarmed his opponent and now held the only weapon. He hoped the man couldn't tell that he didn't know what he was doing. Pei Ke felt the blood running down his right arm, and he could see it dripping on the ground. The pain was getting worse the more he moved.

Pei Ke swung the sword to the left and right numerous times as he closed the distance to his opponent. Every time he swung the broadsword, the opponent moved backwards to get out of range.

On one of his swings, the opponent stepped in and deflected the broadsword to the side, and punched him in the face. Blood started streaming from both nostrils. Pei Ke stumbled backward and the broadsword fell from his hand. The opponent stepped forward and again punched toward Pei Ke's face, but Pei Ke blocked it with the Pi Chuan movement of Hsing-Yi Chuan and followed through with a strike to the man's shoulder. The pain in his arm increased. Pei Ke knew he had to end this quickly or he would die shortly. He stepped in and delivered a ferocious kick to the man's groin. The opponent doubled over in pain as Pei Ke raised his right knee into the man's face. He felt his knee crushing his opponent's nose and blood splattered on his pant leg. He followed this move with a blow to the bridge of the nose. There was a gasp and the man's body went limp. Pei Ke pounced on him ready to deliver a final fatal blow, but he was already dead.

Pei Ke rolled off the man and sat with his head forward. He pressed on Yin Tang acupuncture point to stop the nosebleed. He was exhausted from the ordeal. He looked at the man lying there limp, all the life gone out of him. Blood was spattered on the man's face from where his nose had been broken. Pei Ke looked at his own arm. It was still bleeding.

Many thoughts flooded through his mind, one of which was the realization that the Abbot had set up this attack. The Abbot wanted him killed and this man, whoever he was, was just a tool. Sorrow turned to anger and he stood up, and kicked and cursed the man repeatedly. He cursed the Abbot and he cursed Chen and his men. The angrier he got, the more he kicked and cursed. He finally slumped down on the ground exhausted. He did not know why he was so tired. He felt anger and disgust for what had just happened. The Abbot wanted to kill him. His suspicions were correct about the Abbot.

Finally, he started to calm down. He needed to focus on the current situation. He needed to control his emotions and not let his emotions control him. He needed to plan his next move. After considerable deliberation, he dragged the body into the forest. Walking deeper into the forest, to his surprise he stumbled across two horses tied to a tree, and one of the horses was loaded with supplies. He reasoned that they must have belonged to the man who attacked him. He must have been one of Chen's men who'd come into town, like himself, to get supplies.

He covered the dead body with leaves and debris. He wondered if the man's spirit would understand the circumstances of his death. It was so unnecessary, but it was either kill or be killed. He was grateful he'd learned martial arts from Liu. His teacher had pushed him hard, and many times he wondered why. Now he knew the reason.

He rode one of the assailant's horses and pulled the other one down the path to the stream. He dismounted and washed his face with the cool water of the stream. His nose was still bleeding a little. He again pressed on Yin Tang acupuncture point, and the bleeding stopped shortly thereafter. His arm was still bleeding a little when he tore off a strip of his shirt and applied a tourniquet to his upper arm. Satisfied he had done his best to stop the bleeding his attention turned to the present circumstances.

He debated what to do with the assailant's horses. He could take them with him but decided against that. It would be difficult for him to manage three horses in addition to his own horse. He could leave them where they are but the monks would find them when they came for water, and they would report back to the Abbot. He decided to take the two horses away from the stream. He traveled about two miles west then turned them both loose and returned to where he had left his own two horses.

He quickly mounted his horse and pulled the other one behind him. He headed away from the stream. After a few feet he stopped for a couple of seconds and debated on whether or not to confront the Abbot, but decided it would be best to get the supplies back to Wu's place and leave that to Liu. He was sure the Abbot would deny everything. Liu would know what to do next. Pei Ke rode off, heading south, pulling the horse with the supplies. His arm ached from the wound and his face felt like it was swelling up forcing him to breathe through his mouth.

The Abbot walked from his office to the front of the temple and out on to the street. Pei Ke's horses were gone. The Abbot smiled to himself and walked back into the temple. He went over to the statue of Kuan Yin and bowed to the goddess three times. He then looked down at the floor in front of the statue. He was tempted to remove the stone covering that hid the treasure box, but thought better of it. He had waited this long, he could wait a little while longer and then he would get what he wanted. Chen should have no problem dealing with Liu. He was going to send the monk to relay the information to Chen. Chen would be pleased with the news.

CHAPTER 56

The news from the Abbot was perfect. One down and one to go. It was a stroke of luck that one of his men had been in the village at the same time Liu's student was there. The Abbot had set it up perfectly. Chen knew Liu's student was not an accomplished martial artist; however, he did know something about fighting and one less person to deal with made his mission that much easier.

The Abbot was really a fool if he thought he was going to share the lands and the fortune with him. His father told him it all belonged to the Chen family and no one else. He would deal with the Abbot as soon as he had dealt with the last person standing in his way to get the coveted lands. He briefly wondered where the man was who had taken care of Liu's student. Maybe he was disposing of the body and would soon return. It never crossed his mind that the man would never be returning.

He could not wait for him to return. He had to strike now. He was excited about the fact this conflict was finally going to be over. His father would be proud of him. He could feel the events unfolding in his favor and he needed to get the job done as soon as possible. All his previous efforts were now going to come to fruition.

He and his men prepared to leave immediately. They did not have to take anything other than their weapons. They would all enjoy their rewards shortly after Liu was disposed of and they cheered loudly as they rode out of the compound.

Pei Ke arrived with the supplies and immediately went to Liu and the others to explain what had happened.

"Pei Ke, what happened to you?" asked Liu. "Are you hurt badly? Who did this to you?"

"No, Master I'm fine" said Pei Ke. "These are superficial wounds. My pride is hurt more than my body."

"Well, what happened?"

Liu, Wei Ken De, and the Hu brothers crowded around Pei Ke and listened to his explanation of why his face was swollen, and his shirt was torn and covered with dried blood.

"Master, the monk who reports to the Abbot told me to go to the stream where Chang Song was killed. The Abbot was supposed to meet me there to show me something about his murder, but he never showed up. Instead, when I went there I was attacked by what I suspect was one of Chen's men."

"Are you sure it was one of Chen's men."

"It had to be. The monk and the Abbot were the only ones who knew I was there. The Abbot is in alliance with Chen. I knew we couldn't trust him."

"What happened? Tell me about the fight."

"He had a broadsword and came after me swinging. After a couple of swipes, he cut me in the shoulder, but I managed to take the broadsword away from him. We scuffled for a few minutes. In the end, I killed him."

Liu looked at Wei Ken De and the other men. He did not smile, but the others could see Liu was pleased with what he had heard. His constant instruction with Pei Ke had finally paid off. Pei Ke could now handle himself in a serious life and death altercation. Liu did not have to be so protective anymore.

"What did you do with the body?"

"I took it deep into the forest and covered it up with leaves and debris. I found his horse and pack horse, and took them west a couple of miles and turned them loose. I put his broadsword next to his body. I didn't want to take it in case someone identified it as belonging to him."

Everyone had questions of Pei Ke, even the two Hu brothers who seldom spoke unless asked a direct question. As Pei Ke was explaining the altercation, the men could hear the faint sound of hoofs entering the compound. Wei Ken De went to the window and gasped.

He saw Mei Li riding into the compound along with his trusted servant. He told the others who was coming, and then went to the door and walked outside to greet them. Pei Ke followed, but stopped at the door so he could watch Mei Li without her knowing it. He was suddenly very conscious of his wounds and wondered what she'd think of him. Liu and the Hu brothers waited inside as Liu explained who had arrived.

"Mei Li, I told you to stay at home," said Wei Ken De. "You have no business coming here."

He then turned to his servant.

"I gave you very specific instructions to make sure she stayed at home. Why didn't you stop her from coming here?"

"Master Wei, I tried to stop her. She just got on her horse and left, without me knowing. When I caught up with her, she refused to turn around. The only thing I could have done was to physically restrain her, but that would have meant a struggle between us and I did not believe you would want that. Master, you have to understand my position."

"Father, it's not his fault. Don't blame him he had no choice. He felt he needed to protect me, which I think is ridiculous. I can handle myself. I have come to help fight."

Wei Ken De looked at both of them not knowing what to do. His daughter was head strong, and once she made up her mind to do something, it was virtually impossible to change it. He was upset with his servant, but understood his predicament. At least he came along to make sure that she got here safely. Of course, if anyone had attacked her, they would have been in for quite a surprise.

"Since you both are here, come inside."

"Father, are Pei Ke and Master Liu here?"

"Yes, they are inside with some other men, so come on in and say hello. They will be happy to see you."

Wei Ken De and his servant walked in followed by Mei Li. As she walked in, she glanced at Pei Ke, but walked purposefully to Liu and bowed. He acknowledged the courtesy.

"Mei Li, why have you come here?" asked Liu Bin. "It is not your affair and this fight will be dangerous."

Mei Li looked at Liu for a brief second and debated what she should say to him. Did he or her father really know why she came?

"Master, I came to help you and my father. Pei Ke told us everything, so I know you're outnumbered. Please do not discount me because I'm a woman. I can fight as well as most men. My father has taught me your system of martial arts well."

Liu looked at Wei Ken De. His senior student gave a nod of approval. Liu nodded as well. If Wei Ken De vouched for her, he knew she would be an asset rather than a hindrance and one more person would help even the odds. The Universal Energy was looking after him. He was pleased the way things were developing. He did not want the fight with Chen and his men, but it was the only way to put a halt to the man's evil, and the effect it was having on the people around him.

Pei Ke listened to the discussion, unsure how to feel. He knew firsthand what Chen and his men were capable of and part of him wanted Mei Li as far away from that as possible. But he couldn't deny that he was also happy she was here. He wondered if she was as good in martial arts as she indicated. From what he knew of her, he thought she could probably handle herself. She'd definitely would have the element of surprise, since most men wouldn't anticipate her martial arts abilities. He decided he would do his best to stay close to her and make sure she didn't get hurt. He felt that he needed to protect her.

Mei Li had purposefully ignored everyone else. Now that she had talked with Liu, she turned to Pei Ke and gasped at what she saw.

"Pei Ke what happened to you? Are you hurt badly? Your face is swollen and there is blood on your sleeve and pants."

She walked over to him and touched his sleeve.

"Let me look at your arm."

Embarrassed, he showed her the cut. It was really superficial and the bleeding had stopped, but Mei Li acted like it had practically severed his arm.

"This needs to be cleaned," she said. "I will help you clean it. When did this happen?"

"I was attacked by one of Chen's men while I was in the village getting supplies. He had a broadsword." He paused, then added. "That is how I got cut. His body is hidden back in the forest."

Mei Li looked at Pei Ke and then at her father and Liu Bin then seemed to notice the Hu brothers for the first time.

"Mei Li," said Liu. "You need to meet the Hu brothers. We met them on our travels to Beijing and they have agreed to help us in the upcoming fight with Chen and his men. Both are very skilled, especially with weapons. We are pleased to have them on our side."

Mei Le bowed to the brothers and they acknowledged her courtesy. Then she turned back to Pei Ke.

"Let me see to this wound of yours."

"Wait," Liu said. "I will look at the wound first." He came over to his student. "Pei Ke, is the cut still painful?"

"Master, it is somewhat painful. It doesn't hurt too much if I just let it hang, but when I raise my arm I can feel it." He lifted his arm and winced, but then quickly added. "It's not going to keep me from doing what I need to do."

"Take off your shirt," said Liu.

Liu looked at the wound and then massaged the 'Well Points' on Pei Ke's hand along with some other points above and below the cut.

"How does it feel now?"

"Actually, it feels less tense."

"Hold still and do not move your arm."

Liu rubbed his hands together and then moved his hands to form a cup in close proximity to the wound. Pei Ke felt nothing at first, than he felt energy in the form of continuous waves going from Liu's hands to the area of the wound. Pei Ke felt the whole area relax, and it even seemed that the swelling decreased. Next, Liu simultaneously touched four acupuncture points on Pei Ke's face and the pain in his cheek and nose diminished.

"How do you feel now?"

"Much better," said Pei Ke.

"Pei Ke, my prognosis of this unfortunate accident is that you will live to fight another day. Fortunately or unfortunately, that may be sooner than you think. You are fine. You just need to get cleaned up."

"Mei Li."

"Yes, Master."

"Help Pei Ke. Down the hallway, in one of the bedrooms there are some of Wu's shirts. Get one and then get some water and strips of clean cloth and take care of his wound."

As Mei Li turned and headed for the hallway, Pei Ke also started to leave.

"Pei Ke, you stay here."

Liu waited until Mei Li was out of hearing range.

"Wei Ken De, is she ready to fight and is she capable of handling herself against these men?"

"She and I have sparred together continuously, but she has never had to fight someone she did not know. Still, I think she will be able to handle someone so long as he is not too big. I'm afraid she may be intimidated by an attacker's size. And she has not had the opportunity to fight multiple attackers."

"May I interrupt?" said Pei Ke, and without waiting for an answer, he continued. "I will stay close to her and make sure no harm is done to her."

Pei Ke then looked directly into Wei Ken De's eyes. He remembered the first time he'd met Wei Ken De and how intimidated he'd felt. There was none of that now. He knew Wei Ken De was senior to him and definitely more accomplished, but he had now asserted his position within Liu's inner door students. Even though he was not an equal, he was included within the circle.

There was only a slight nod from Wei Ken De as Mei Li came back into the room with water, strips of cloth, and a shirt.

As the group discussed the upcoming situation with Chen, Mei Li looked closely at the wound. For a moment, Pei Ke thought she was actually looking at him and not the wound. To cover his embarrassment, he looked into her eyes. She blushed a little, then took a damp cloth and busied herself cleaning the wound.

She was amazed at how muscular he was and that there was not a bit of fat on his body. No doubt, he had not always looked this good. It must have been the rigorous training Liu put him through that made his body so rock hard and strong. He was of good stock. She looked over at her father, who was staring at her, then she turned her head and continued the process of cleaning and bandaging Pei Ke's wound. It was imperative that she talk with Master Liu as soon as possible. There was no way she was going to let Liu and Pei Ke go off on another jaunt without having her say as to her future. She wanted to be part of Pei Ke's life, and she wanted to believe that he had thought only of her while he had been gone.

"Mei Li, are you finished putting him back together?" Liu said. "He is not so delicate that you have to pamper him."

Mei Li blushed again.

"Master, he is ready to go."

"Fine, we are going to go now to my ancestral home. If I am correct, we should find that they are not there. Chen is rather impatient, and I suspect that he and his men are traveling this way as we speak. If not, and they are still at my home, we will make other plans. But for now, we assume they will be coming here and we need to leave.

"There were some swords and broadswords left behind from the massacre so pick one and let's get moving. Pei Ke, do you have my sack."

"Yes, Master."

Liu quickly led the way out the door followed by Wei Ken De, the two Hu brothers, and Wei Ken De's servant. Pei Ke started to move toward the door. When the others were out the door, Mei Li took hold of his good arm, and raised herself on her toes and kissed him on the cheek. Then she quickly stepped in front of him and out the door.

Liu got to his horse and was about to mount when he suddenly stopped and headed back to the house.

"Wait for me. I forgot to do something. It will only take a minute or two and we can be on our way."

Once inside he found some ink, a calligraphy brush, and a large piece of rice paper. He wrote on the paper and put it on the floor just inside the door. He put an ink stone on the top edge of the paper to keep it in place and then went back outside to his horse.

CHAPTER 57

Chen and his men were guiding their horses south through the center of the village. The Abbot was inside the temple at the back and out of visual range of the street. He could see them, but they could not see him. He watched as the men rode past. This was going to be the end of the conflict. There was no way Liu by himself, was going to be able to defeat Chen and his men.

He briefly thought about joining Chen's group, but being a cautious man he decided not to. It was best that he not be seen taking sides in this matter. After all, it was not a temple matter, but a matter between two families. He could wait.

Liu and his fellow martial artists headed north, keeping to the west of the village. Liu did not want to run into Chen anywhere along the road. He did not know where Chen was at that precise moment, but guessed he was somewhere on the road to Wu's place. Liu could feel evilness off to the east, and on one occasion, he sensed evil following them.

His goal was to be in his ancestral home when Chen attacked so he could honestly tell everyone he was defending himself and his property. Liu and his party traveled north through the forest and farmland areas for quite some distance until Liu felt Chen was now either in the village or south of the village. He guided them back to the main road and continued their journey north to his ancestral home.

———————————————

Chen and his men were five minutes from the Wu compound. He stopped and considered how he was going to initiate the encounter.

Chen pointed to one of his men. "Go to the house. See if Liu Bin is there, then come right back. I expect Liu will be there, but I do not want to attack the place only to find that it is a trap."

One of his men rode off ahead of the group. Half an hour later, he returned with a piece of rice paper. Chen read it then swore. The note said:

> *Exceptional results can be achieved with small forces.*
> *—Sun Tzu*

> *With all your men, you cannot defeat me. I have outwitted you again. You are a fool. I knew you were coming. The Abbot has betrayed you. Give it up and go away before you are killed. I go to be with my family. I am but one man. The Universal Energy will protect me.*

"He is only one man," said Chen. "He cannot win this fight." He turned to his men. "Everyone will receive their reward once Liu Bin is dead. Now get some rest. We're on our way at first light."

———————————————

Liu saw that the gate was open as he and the others rode up to his ancestral home. He distinctly remembered that Pei Ke had locked it when they were previously there. The only thing he could think of was that it must have been Chen and his men who failed to close it. Chen had been in a hurry to leave or he felt that it was not necessary to lock it.

Pei Ke closed and locked the gate after they entered. Liu assigned rotating guards to watch the compound for the night. Retiring for the night, Liu felt no evilness in close proximity to where they were, and anticipated no response from Chen that evening.

As he lay in his bed, he was deep in thought about the strategies he had learned from the works of Sun Tzu and he wanted to make no mistakes in this altercation. His thoughts turned to his family who had died from Chen's evilness. He felt nothing but sadness and anger. Why did they have to die, especially the children? They were so innocent. Why did Hua Yee, his true heir, have to die on the mountain?

Sleep did not come easy for Pei Ke. He was restless, thinking about the fight that was certain to come the next day. He needed to be brave and do his part in putting an end to Chen's brutality. He prayed to Kuan Yin to give him the strength, both mental and physical, to do what was needed. Just before he fell asleep, he thought of the untimely death of Hua Yee. He also thought of his visit to Beijing. He would like to go back there again. It would be a good place for him to gain more experience before he became a doctor. He would have to speak with Liu Bin when this nasty business with Chen was over.

Mei Li was worried that her impulsive move with Pei Ke would send the wrong message to him. As she pondered her brave and impulsive act, she decided it had been the right thing to do under the circumstances. Her mother would have been horrified and she would have been disciplined severely, but she had to send a message to Pei Ke, and kissing him on the cheek was the most effective and emotionally strong message she could think of at the moment.

She needed to talk with Liu Bin. Hopefully, he would understand and be on her side, and help convince her father that Pei Ke was the one for her.

Wei Ken De thought of his daughter. Had he been correct to bring her up to be so independent? It was not the custom of society, but she needed to be able to fend for herself in this world if she was to inherit his business and estate. Maybe a strong husband would also help.

CHAPTER 58

One of Chen's men walked into the temple and went immediately to the Abbot's outer office.

"Where is the Abbot?"

"He is busy. May I help you," said one of the monks who helped the Abbot?

"No, I need to see the Abbot. I can wait for a minute or two."

The monk went into the Abbot's office and a few minutes later, he emerged.

"You may go in now."

The man walked in and closed the door.

"I have told Chen numerous times that he and his men must not come to the temple," said the Abbot. "Each time you come, there is more reason for others to be suspicious about my activities."

"I have a message from Chen."

"What is it?"

"He says he now has the amulets. Do you want him to come to the temple for you to look at them, or do you want to meet him someplace?"

"Where is he now?"

"He is outside of the village in the forest on the east side. He wanted me to tell you that he has what he needs now. He wants to know the significance of the amulets. Should I bring him here to see you?"

"No, no. That is not necessary. I will go with you. Let me get one of the monks to go with us."

"Chen never mentioned bringing someone else."

"This monk has helped me in this matter, and I trust him to be discrete."

"Are you sure you don't want Chen to come here?"

"No, that is not necessary. Let me get the monk and we can go."

That night Chen looked at the three amulets in his possession. He had taken one from the dead body of Hua Yee, one from the servant boy he had killed, and now he had the one from the Abbot. There was one missing and Liu must have it. He tried to understand the writings on the amulets, but realized that unless he had all four of them he could not make much sense out of the puzzle.

He would wear the three amulets around his neck for safe keeping and when Liu was dead he would add the fourth coin and hopefully solve the mystery of why everyone safeguarded these amulets. The coins had something to do with the treasure. Maybe it gave directions to where the treasure was located.

The Abbot and the monk who went with him never returned to the temple. Chen buried them in a nondescript grave. Only Liu Bin stood in his way now to secure the lands and any treasure. He looked forward to being victorious in the struggle he and his father had been involved with for so long. The lands would finally be his and his father would be proud of him. Liu had killed his father and he was going to kill Liu.

CHAPTER 59

iu once again felt an uneasiness in the Universal Energy. It was similar in nature to the uneasiness he felt when he observed those evil eyes, which had followed him for so many months. Something had just happened which was significant to him regarding his upcoming fight with Chen and his men. He did not know what it was, but this was one more indication that everything preceding today was now coming to a final solution. He looked forward to the solution and was sure he was going to be victorious. Liu gathered everyone around him.

"I hope you all slept well last night," said Liu. "I want to thank each of you again for being here today to help me resolve this problem. I am confident we will come out of this victorious. I believe Chen and his men will attack either today or tonight. We need to have a coordinated response to whatever takes place. I am certain that Chen does not know that any of you are here and he is expecting this to be quite easy." Liu smiled grimly. "If we plan correctly, we will give him a nasty surprise."

"What is the plan?" asked one of the Hu brothers.

"Chen likes to attack with stealth and under the cover of darkness. He will probably arrive sometime between midnight and first light. He is familiar with this compound, and he will assume I am sleeping in one of the bedrooms in the main house. He will have one man go over the wall to open the main gate, and since he is very cautious, he will send one of his men in first to make sure it isn't a trap.

Their primary objective is to kill me. His men are following him because he is their leader. Once Chen is dead, they will realize that there is no way they will ever get any benefit from continuing the fight. Killing Chen is our main objective, but we must do it with a plan."

As they sat down to drink tea, Liu explained what his plan was for the upcoming attack. There were a couple of questions as well as suggestions on how the plan was going to work and who was going to do what. After an hour of discussion, they all agreed that they had orchestrated the best plan for the upcoming attack. They drank their tea as Liu shared more information about what he and Pei Ke did on their trip to Beijing. During the conversation one of the Hu brothers asked.

"Will you or Pei Ke be coming back with us to the village when this is over? The villagers really respect you for your martial arts ability and, especially, for your expertise in acupuncture and herbs. Of course, from what we hear from the villagers, there are a number of young ladies there who have their eyes on Pei Ke. We understand there is one in particular who is very interested in him. She has even made him meals."

Both men laughed. Pei Ke was caught totally off guard by the comment. He started to blush. Mei Li was caught off guard just as much as Pei Ke. She looked at him and then looked at her father and then at Liu. Liu thought for a second and decided on what he wanted to say.

"There are too many variables for me to entertain a decision at this minute. Pei Ke has been with me for some time now and, of course, he needs to make his own decision. From what the villagers have told me, he is more than welcome there at any time. In fact, it would be a perfect opportunity for him."

"Well, Pei Ke," said one of the Hu brothers. "What are you going to do when this is finished? We will be going back as soon as it is over. You could ride with us."

Pei Ke looked around the table. What was he to say and at such an awkward moment? He looked at Mei Li, then her father, and then back to Mei Li. He could see the questioning in her eyes, but he couldn't say what he wanted to say in front of everyone.

"I agree with Teacher," he said finally. There are too many variables. Let's get this unfortunate upcoming attack over with."

"You may want to make a decision soon," said one of the men. "These ladies are not going to wait on you forever. From what we hear, you were the main attraction, and I think when you return you'll have your pick of whomever you want. The girls and their mothers will stumble all over themselves trying to gain favor with you."

Mei Li looked at her father. Their eyes met and he saw the message in her gaze. It was a message of pleading and firmness. Wei Ken De looked at Liu. He could not tell if there was a smile on his face or not. There was silence at the table as everyone drank their tea. Mei Li and Pei Ke looked briefly at each other. This did not go unnoticed by everyone, especially Wei Ken De.

Chen and his men were camped close to the road leading to the Liu compound. They were close enough they could transverse the distance to the compound in a very short time, but far enough away that no one would know they were there.

The time for the attack was drawing near as Chen brought his men together in a circle and explained how they were going to do it. He did not expect anyone to be there except Liu. However, they needed to be careful just in case he had recruited one or two men from the village. If so, they should not be much of a deterrent as they were only villagers and not fighters. He cautioned them on the Liu's martial arts expertise

CHAPTER 60

Early in the morning, a couple of hours before the sun rose, Chen positioned his men in front of the large gate. As he had expected, the gate was locked. He remembered leaving the compound with the gate closed but not locked. He sent one of his men to climb over the wall as he had done before.

Liu watched through one of the windows of the main house as the faint light from the moon illuminated the open compound. He watched as someone climbed over the west wall and dropped into the compound. After a few seconds, the man walked toward the main gate. He opened the gate and two men cautiously joined him in the compound.

The three of them saw one horse tethered to the hitch at the main house. Since they had been here before, they knew their way around the compound and house. Liu saw their confidence rise as they assumed that Liu was really here, by himself, and was going to make his last stand at his ancestral home. As the three men approached the house, Liu moved away from the window to one of the bedrooms. He had purposely left the main bedroom empty as he positioned everyone in strategic places in the house. This meant the attackers would have to go from room to room to find Liu.

The first of Chen's men slowly opened the door and walked into the main sitting room, followed closely by the other two. Once they were in the house, Chen himself and six men entered the compound. He assigned two of the six men to guard the front entrance to make sure Liu did not escape.

Once he and the rest of his men were inside, he signaled that they should start their search. The night before, he'd drawn a diagram of the house in the dirt and assigned two-man teams to enter each bedroom. They were to position themselves outside the doors and, at his command, rush into the bedrooms all at the same time. One of the groups was bound to find Liu. They were to kill him immediately if they found him. Chen and one of the men would work their way down the hallway from one room to the other to make sure that everything went as planned. They were going to help as much as possible when they came to each room and serve as a back up to the team that discovered Liu.

Liu had done the same thing. However, he assigned no one to the first bedroom. The two Hu brothers were to be in the second bedroom. He was going to be in the third bedroom with Mei Li. Wei Ken De and Pei Ke were going to be in the fourth bedroom. Initially, Wei Ken De had objected to this, but Liu reminded him that he would fight better if he did not have to worry about his daughter. Reluctantly, Wei Ken De agreed and the trap was set. Pei Ke also wanted to be with Mei Li, but Liu was insistent on the arrangement. If no one entered, their respective rooms, then they were to immediately go and help whoever needed help.

Wei Ken De's servant was to go out the back door when Chen arrived and hide in the shadows until all of Chen's men were inside the compound. When he heard the fighting, he was to shut the gate and kill anyone who tried to escape.

As soon as the door opened and Chen's men entered a room, the defenders were going to rush them, shouting at the top of their voices in an effort to cause confusion and anxiety.

As he had done before, and as his father had done before him, Chen gave the signal and his men burst into their assigned rooms and quickly headed for the beds.

Those who burst into the first bedroom found no one, but immediately they heard shouts and screams coming from the other bedrooms.

Two of Chen's men rushed into the second bedroom with their swords in hand, ready to attack. They were immediately met by the Hu brothers, who charged forward. The darkness in the room was to the advantage of the defenders. The clash of metal against metal echoed in the room as the defenders quickly turned the situation to their favor. One of Chen's men died almost as soon as he entered the room. The other died seconds later. They were no match for two accomplished martial artists. The two brothers dragged the bodies away from the door and went into the hallway where they met up with the two intruders from the first room.

Wei Ken De and Pei Ke waited for the door to open. The two who entered their room were both accomplished martial artists and knew fully well how to handle weapons. Wei Ken De charged the first one and after the man's initial surprise, their fight moved from the doorway to the middle of the room, allowing the second man to rush in and attack Pei Ke.

From the first crossing of the swords, Wei Ken De knew that he was a far superior swordsman than his opponent. Pei Ke, however, felt clumsy with his weapon and knew he didn't stand a chance unless he closed the distance and grabbed hold of the opponent's sword.

The second of Chen's men through the door quickly sized up the situation and took one quick swing at Pei Ke, forcing him to backup. The man sneered contemptuously at Pei Ke, than turned his attention to Wei Ken De who was obviously the bigger threat.

What was to be an easy victory for Wei Ken De now turned into a fight for his life. He could easily handle one of them, but it was nearly impossible for him to handle two of them at the same time in the darkened room. Wei Ken De deflected the two sword attacks. He was backing up when the second man moved four feet to his right to attack from the side, while the first man attacked from the front. For a moment, the second man's back was in front of Pei Ke.

Pei Ke leaped forward and swung his sword with both hands at the second man's right knee. The sword cut completely through the joint, muscles, and tendons, severing the man's leg. The assailant screamed as he collapsed to the floor.

Pei Ke then lifted his sword above his head and sliced downward against the first man's shoulder cutting deep into bone and tissue knocking the sword from the assailant's hand.

The first man screamed loudly as Wei Ken De then thrust his sword deep into his opponent's chest. The tip of the sword punctured the heart. He died instantly.

Pei Ke turned to the second assailant, who was flailing on the floor, and finished him with a swift stab to the chest.

Pei Ke heard Mei Li screaming and quickly ran out the bedroom and down the hallway to the fourth bedroom. He entered to find Liu and one of Chen's men in a clashing dual of swords.

Mei Li was backed against the wall deflecting vicious sword blows. As Pei Ke came in, her assailant changed the direction of his attack in mid-swing, knocking the sword from her hand. He then raised his sword for a swift, downward blow to her head. Pei Ke bellowed and lunged forward blocking the downward swing with his sword, saving her life.

The man's sword swung wide away from Mei Li, but cut across Pei Ke's chest. Wei Ken De roared in on Pei Ke's heels and without hesitation killed the man with a quick slice to his throat. Gurgling sounds signaled his demise as blood spurted forth from his neck and mouth.

Liu finished the man he was fighting with a stab to the man's abdomen and then to his head. Liu and Wei Ken De looked at Pei Ke, who was covered in blood from his wound and from the men he'd killed.

"Mei Li, take care of Pei Ke," said Liu.

Liu and Wei Ken De went into the hallway. They saw the Hu brothers down the hallway checking the other rooms. Liu and Wei Ken De turned to see Chen standing in the hallway with one of his men. Liu and Wei Ken De ran down the hallway toward Chen. Wei Ken De immediately attacked Chen's companion and the man proved to be no match for his expertise. The death was swift and almost painless.

"Wei Ken De, check outside," said Liu.

Outside, the two men Chen had left behind in the courtyard heard the commotion and ran toward the locked gate. Wei Ken De ran outside and saw his servant blocking their escape. He ran as fast as he could to the gate. The two attackers were no match for Wei Ken De and his servant. Like the others, they died on the spot.

Wei Ken De hurried back to be with Liu, and the servant stayed at the gate to prevent anyone else from escaping.

"Liu, I am going to kill you now," said Chen.

"Chen, you and your father have committed the most heinous of crimes against my family. First, you killed my brother and his family, and then you killed Wu and tried to kill my niece. You will not leave here alive. Even if you somehow manage to kill me, one of these men will kill you. You have no way out. You are a dead man."

Chen charged Liu with a shriek, swinging wildly. Liu stepped to one side, decreasing the surface area under attack and deflecting the oncoming sword. Liu then swung his own sword toward Chen's head. Chen blocked the attack then stepped to the right and thrust straight at Liu's abdomen. Liu sidestepped the thrust and blocked the attack.

Wei Ken De quickly walked into the sitting room relieved to see that his teacher was ok. He was going to help Liu when Liu waved him aside.

Chen pressed the attack with repeated thrusts and swings and each time, Liu was a half second ahead of him. This continued for a couple of minutes with Chen constantly pressing forward, and Liu successfully countering each move.

Liu saw that with each attack, Chen became less accurate with his thrusts and his breathing became more labored. Wei Ke De watched and wondered why his teacher was not pressing the attack. Chen was no match for Liu. The fight was lopsided. Why didn't Liu just finish it and be done with Chen? He then realized that Liu was just playing with Chen.

As Chen continued his attacks, Wei Ken De analyzed each attack and the defense that Liu used to counter it. This went on with Chen attacking and Liu defending. As he watched, Wei Ken De suddenly realized that he was no longer watching a sword fight, as desperate as it all seemed. Instead, Liu was giving him a personal lesson on how to use a sword. He watched closely as Chen became frustrated with his inability to penetrate Liu's defenses. Wei Ken De hoped that the fight would go on forever. What a lesson in swordsmanship. This was better than anything Liu had previously taught him.

Chen was totally out of breath, but he made one last attempt at pressing the attack. He held onto his sword with both hands and swung it wildly back and forth in a figure eight pattern. He lunged at Liu, but Liu blocked the sword and it fell from Chen's hands. Liu turned in a complete circle after deflecting the attack and with one fast swing of his sword decapitated his opponent. Chen's head fell to the floor, followed by the thump of his body.

Liu walked over to the head and kicked it as hard as he could. It bounced against the wall and rolled back in front of Liu. Liu spit on the head and then spit on Chen's decapitated body.

He bent down and opened Chen's shirt and there he found three amulets, which he took and put around his neck. When he searched the body further, he found three pieces of paper. He read them briefly, then and put them inside his shirt. He found the paper given to Chen's father by the warlord, awarding him custody of the land. He opened the scroll and read it.

When he finished reading it, a rush of energy swirled around the room. Liu felt it, and he was sure Wei Ken De felt it. It was a cleansing, as if the negative energy, which had existed for so long, departed. It was a relief for Liu. He hadn't realized how much that energy had negatively affected him until the burden was lifted. He was finally free of the evilness that had pursued him. The energy of the dark side came from Chen, and the evilness of the eyes belonged to the evilness of Chen. Sadness descended upon him as he realized that his family was no longer a part of his life, and he was the last of the Liu family, as he knew it.

"Is everyone ok?" asked Liu.

"We are fine," said one of the Hu brothers.

"Where are Mei Li and Pei Ke?"

Everyone walked back to the bedroom where Pei Ke and Mei Li were left behind. Pei Ke was lying on the bed. His shirt was off and blood was running down the front of his chest.

"Master, I can't get the bleeding to stop," sobbed Mei Li. "What should I do? Please Master, help! I don't want him to die."

Tears rolled down her cheeks as she looked at Liu.

"Squeeze the wound together where it is bleeding and compress it lightly. Maybe that will help."

Mei Li did as instructed and the bleeding stopped. She released the compression and it started bleeding again.

"Mei Li, you are going to have to hold the compression for some time until the bleeding stops. Can you do this?"

"Yes, Master. I will do anything to help. Is he going to be all right? Is he going to live? He's not going to die, is he?"

"Pei Ke, how do you feel?" asked Liu.

"The cut hurts, but it isn't any worse than the cut on my arm. I just feel a little weak and tired."

"You have lost some blood and you are tired from the mental and physical exertion," said Liu. "You will be fine as soon as the bleeding stops and you get some food in you. I will prepare some herbs for you to build up your strength.

"Pei Ke, do you remember which herb to use to stop bleeding?"

Wei Ken De chuckled.

"Yes, Master," Pei Ke said groggily. "It is Yin Nan Bi Yao."

"Then maybe you should tell Mei Le what to do to help you."

"Yes Master."

Liu and the others left the room as Pei Ke began to instruct Mei Li about the herb and how it works. She went to find the sack that Pei Ke always carried and found the little bottle that had the powder. She carefully followed his instructions and then squeezed the wound and compressed it and held it in place. The bleeding stopped shortly thereafter.

"Pei Ke, what are you and Liu going to do now that Chen is dead?" asked Mei Li. They were alone and she desperately wanted to talk to him. He needed to know how she felt about him. She yearned he would say those words that would solidify their relationship.

"I don't know. I am his student, and I'll do whatever he wants me to do. I have learned so much about acupuncture while we were in Beijing, but I realize I have only scratched the surface. There is so much to learn. The more I learn, the more I realize what I don't know, and the more I want to learn."

Mei Li looked at Pei Ke and then looked at the door to make sure no one was watching. She hesitated for a brief second, and then lifted up his hand and quickly kissed the back of it. She looked into his eyes and smiled. As she held onto his hand, the most daring of thoughts went through her mind. She wanted so much for him to realize how she felt, that she would do just about anything to convey the message. At that moment, Liu walked into the bedroom and looked at Pei Ke and Mei Li. She put his hand back on the bed and stood up. Liu saw she was blushing. He pretended not to notice.

"I see he is still alive. I would like to talk with everyone for a few minutes."

Liu walked out of the room, and Mei Li helped Pei Ke to get up, and they both followed him into the main room.

"How is the wound," asked Liu. "Has the bleeding stopped?"

"Master, the bleeding has stopped," said Pei Ke.

Liu looked around the room.

"Where are the Hu brothers?" asked Liu.

"We are here. We have been checking the other rooms to make sure that no one else is hiding."

"Good," said Liu. "Is everyone alright?"

Everyone looked at Pei Ke.

"He is alright," said Liu. "He only has a few wounds that he can later brag about."

Liu hesitated before speaking.

"We need to dispose of the bodies. I do not want to bury them on this land. This land belongs to my family, and I do not want to desecrate it with the bad energy these bodies represent. We need to take them into the mountains away from this area and bury them together in an unmarked grave."

"There is a cart in the barn. We can hitch one of their horses to the cart, load the bodies on the cart, and take them away at first light. Right now, I want to get them out of my house and away from us, and particularly away from me.

"Wei Ke De, please take one of their horses and go to the barn and hitch it to the cart. The rest of us will drag the bodies outside and wait for the cart. Mei Li I would like you to get some water and clean the blood from the floor and walls. There are some lanterns in the kitchen area that will help you to see. Pei Ke is weak from the loss of blood and should not exert himself. However, he can hold the lantern for you.

"Let's get this started and finished before the end of the day."

Late that afternoon, they arrived back at Liu's ancestral home. They had buried the bodies in a remote area of the mountains facing away from the

Liu lands. They put no markers on the gravesite and all the bodies were buried together in one mass grave. No one would ever come to pay them respect. The men Chen had recruited over the various months had paid the price for their greed and dishonesty. Liu was sad about the needless deaths but relieved that he could now live in peace.

They could see the exhaustion in each other's faces as they dismounted from their horses and walked into the house. Wei Ken De took the horses to the barn and prepared them for the evening. When he returned to the house, everyone was drinking tea and Mei Li was preparing some vegetables and rice for the group.

"We do not have too much to eat," said Mei Li.

"Anything will do," said the Hu brothers in unison.

"Tomorrow we'll go into the village and get whatever supplies we need," said Liu.

As they started to eat, Liu cleared his throat and looked at each of them.

"Tonight, we all need to get plenty of sleep. I want to thank each of you for what you did here today on my behalf. I will always be indebted to you, and if I can repay you in any way, please do not hesitate to ask me."

They finished their meal in silence, each of them too tired to talk. All they wanted was some food, tea, and a nice comfortable bed to sleep in. After dinner, they were finishing their tea in the sitting area when Wei Ken De stood up.

"Father," said Mei Li. "Before you retire for the night may I visit with you for a few minutes?"

"Unless it is life threatening, let it wait till tomorrow. I am tired and I want to go to bed."

He bowed to Liu and the others and left the room.

"Master Liu, may I speak with you," asked Mei Li.

"We are all tired. Please leave it for tomorrow. I will be happy to visit with you and answer any of your questions at that time."

Liu stood up and left the room. Mei Li looked at Pei Ke. He was sound asleep.

"He needs to get some sleep," said one of the Hu brothers. "His wound isn't serious, but he lost a lot of blood and his body needs to recuperate. We will take him and put him in bed."

Mei Li went to bed, but she could not let go of the thought of her father and Liu being so tired they could not take time to talk to her. She hated being ignored like that, and as she lay in bed, she heard first one then another of the men snoring. At first, it was light and didn't bother her; however, it grew to a crescendo, each one taking their own turn making ever more noise.

She wondered if Pei Ke snored, but she herself was too tired to go and find out. She eventually fell asleep, thinking of Pei Ke. She wondered what it would be like to be married to him. She was sure he would be a good husband and treat her with tenderness, respect, and dignity, even if he did snore.

CHAPTER 61

The next morning, Liu and Wei Ken De were up as the sun inched its way over the mountains. It was a cool but beautiful morning. After finishing their Qi Gong exercises, they sat in the sitting room drinking tea as the rest of the group slept.

"Master, I hope the death of Chen has ended your torment. It is sad that so many of your family died for the greed of just one person."

"It was not just one person," said Liu. "It started with the father and passed on to the son. With his death, it is over and we all can return to a normal life."

"Master, what will you do now?" asked Wei Ken De.

"The Hu brothers need to get back to the village. I promised the village elders they would return as soon as possible to fulfill the rest of their contract. When they wake up, I will pay them and they can decide what they want to do.

"As for the rest of us, I think we should rest here for a few days and enjoy the peacefulness of this wonderful valley. It will give us all time to think about what we need to do. I would like for the four of us to ride through the valley, so you all can see the extent of the land.

"At some point, however, I need to go into the village, and I would like for the three of you to join me. You know the story of the amulets, and what they represent, but you do not know their true value. We will visit the temple and retrieve the box that was put there by my father for safekeeping."

"What about the Abbot? Don't you suspect he had something to do with Chen?"

"I believe the Abbot was honest until he realized if all my family was killed, this land and its treasure would be available to anyone. Like many other people in positions of authority, the idea of money and what it can do clouded his judgment, and when the opportunity presented itself, he took advantage of it. Basically, it is greed and opportunity. He wanted something he did not have and there was an opportunity for him to get it with little or no effort on his part. Unfortunately, for him, there is little to no honor among thieves, and I am sure Chen killed him just before he attacked us."

"Master, may I ask you a question?" asked Wei Ken De.

"Of course," said Liu.

"As you know, Mei Li has been asking me about her future."

"Yes, she probably wanted to discuss it last night."

"Yes, but it was not the time to do so. I think it would be appropriate for Pei Ke and her to get married. Do you agree?"

"Pei Ke was thinking about Hua Yee and Mei Li. I do not think he had made up his mind one way or the other. Of course, both girls had their minds made up and were both interested in him. As far as I know, neither one of them knew the other had an interest in Pei Ke. Unfortunately, my niece is dead. When Pei Ke and I were in the village to the east, there were a number of mothers who took an immediate interest in him. They were not subtle and even Pei Ke understood their intention. I do not think he has any interest in them. The question is what does Pei Ke want to do?

"He has many choices. I personally feel he needs to study martial arts from someone else for a while. You would be the most obvious person since you would be just a continuation of what I have already taught him but from your own perspective. The question is would you be willing to teach him. Also would you want him as an addition to your family?"

Wei Ken De looked thoughtfully out the window at the rising sun.

"During the fight, he actually saved both my life and Mei Li's life. For that, I am indebted to him. I think you might want to talk to him after you have decided what you intend to do. Are you going to stay here with your ancestral lands or are you going to go back to the temple to the south? Your decision may have a bearing on what Pei Ke wants to do.

"I suspect Mei Li is enthralled with him. She needs someone who has the same interests as she. Because of the way my wife and I trained her she would not be comfortable in a highly submissive role. It is unfortunate she is the only child and there were no boys to take over my business. She will be the one to take over when I pass on unless there is someone who would be willing to join in with her."

As Liu and Wei Ken De were talking, they heard the shuffling of feet and the Hu brothers sauntered into the sitting room.

"Is there anything else you need from us?" asked one of the brothers.

"No, you have done well, and I am indebted to you both," said Liu.

"We shall be on our way then. The sooner we get started, the sooner we will get back to the village. The villagers will be wondering what has happened to us."

"You are welcome to stay with us," said Liu.

"No, we discussed it last night before we went to sleep. We need to return to the village. We're going to leave this morning. In fact if it is alright with you we would like to leave now."

"It is fine with me. I will walk you out to the barn and we can talk while you saddle your horses."

Liu and the two brothers walked to the barn. As they saddled their horses, Liu took some coins from his pocket and gave them to the two men.

"This is more than we agreed," said one of the brothers.

"You have done me a much needed service and you both are honest and decent men. Hopefully, in the not too distant future, we will meet again. Please know you both are welcome in my home at any time."

"Is there anything you want us to convey to the elders of the village?"

"Yes, tell them one day we might meet again. You might also want to indirectly mention that Pei Ke is now committed to a young lady here in this village. It is not right for that mother and young girl to keep hoping he will return."

The men laughed, then rode out the gate and up the road to the top of the mountain and over the summit on the way back to the village. Liu watched them ride away. Then he walked back to the main house and entered through the front door. Mei Li and Pei Ke were up and having some tea with Wei Ken De.

"The Hu brothers have departed. They wanted to get back as soon as possible. I have changed my mind. I would like for all of us to go into the village this morning."

Liu Bin, Pei Ke, and Wei Ken De's servant were on horseback while Wei Ken De and Mei Li rode in the carriage. They stopped in front of the temple. As was discussed the previous evening, the servant was to continue back to Wei Ken De's home to look after the estate. As the servant rode away, they hitched their horses, and walked into the temple and went directly to the Abbot's office.

"Master Liu, have you seen the Abbot?" asked the assistant Abbot. "We haven't seen him in a couple of days. In fact, I was going to send someone out to your place to see if he was there."

"No, none of us have seen him. Do you have any clues as to where he might have gone?"

"He left here with one of the other monks and we haven't seen him since. He didn't tell anyone where he was going. It really seems strange. We're afraid something has happened to him."

"I do not know where he is. Do you want me to search up north? We will be going back after we get some supplies and finish our business here."

"Yes, please."

"I assume that in the Abbot's absence you are in charge."

"Yes."

"Are you aware my father left some valuables here at the temple?"

"Yes, but that's all that I know."

"I would like to collect those items now."

The man looked nervously around.

"Master Liu, I have no idea where they're stored."

"I know where everything is located, and I would like to take the items with me. If the Abbot were here, I would be telling him I am taking them, but he is not here now. If the Abbot returns tell him I was here."

"Yes, Master."

Pei Ke, Wei Ken De, Mei Li and the assistant Abbot followed Liu as he walked into the main temple area. Liu directed them to the statue of Kuan Yin. Liu knelt down in front of the statue. He motioned for Wei Ken De to help him. Together, with their fingers wedged between two flat stones, they lifted one, revealing an open space with a metal box inside. They lifted the heavy metal box from its hiding place. It made a sharp metallic sound as it touched the floor. Liu and Wei Ken De carefully replaced the stone covering and made sure there was no evidence that someone had lifted it out of the floor.

"Master, I never knew there was a hiding place here," said the assistant Abbot. "No one would ever guess this hiding place existed. Many have stood or kneeled on this spot when they've prayed to Kuan Yin. I guess the Abbot was the only one who knew about it."

"Yes, and I would like for the hiding place to remain secret," said Liu.

"Yes, Master. Your secret is safe with me."

"I am going to take this box with me now and I may return it in the next couple of days," said Liu.

"I will tell the Abbot when he returns," said the assistant Abbot.

"Yes, hopefully he will return soon," said Liu.

They took the box out to the carriage. Then, they finished their activities in the village and went back to Liu's ancestral home.

CHAPTER 62

They arrived back at Liu's compound late in the afternoon. Wei Ken De set the metal box on the floor of the sitting room. Pei Ke, Wei Ken De, and Mei Li watched as Liu studied the box. He had not seen it for many years and its sight here in his boyhood home brought back wonderful memories of a happy family.

His father had the wisdom and insight to keep valuable information hidden from others who might misuse it. Liu knew what was in the box, but needed to reassure himself that the contents were still intact.

Liu took the three amulets from around his neck. He detached the cord from the amulets, and put them on the floor next to the box.

"Pei Ke I need the amulet you have around your neck."

Pei Ke took the amulet from around his neck, detached the cord, and put it on the floor next to the other amulets.

"This box was constructed of the strongest metal available. As you can see, there are no hinges, knobs, or handles. The box can be opened when the four amulets are inserted into four separate slots, one on each side of the box. Notice that each amulet has a slightly different shape. When put together they form a perfect circle."

Liu took the four amulets and arranged them on the floor to form a circle. Once he had arranged them, everyone saw that there were Chinese characters etched on the surface of the amulets.

"Master," said Mei Li. "Once you align the four amulets correctly the characters indicate the Five Elements of Metal, Water, Wood, Fire, and Earth. And there are other writings on the amulets."

"Yes, that is correct. You will also notice that none of the amulets is exactly alike. The edges are different for each of them. This way we will know if the four amulets are the correct amulets. To open the box, each amulet is inserted into a slot on the side of the box. If an amulet is inserted into the wrong slot, nothing will happen.

"When an amulet is inserted into the correct slot, there will be a slight click taking place as a lever is released inside the box. This will not happen if the edges of the amulet are incorrect or the amulet is inserted into the wrong slot. The levers release the cover of the box so that the cover can be slid to the right, thus opening the box."

"Master, how do you know which amulet goes into which slot?" asked Pei Ke.

Wei Ken De and Mei Li watched in fascination as Liu explained to Pei Ke the workings and intricacies of the metal box.

"If you try to slide an amulet into the wrong slot it will not go all the way into the slot. If you try to force it into the slot, the amulet will break and it will be almost impossible to open the box without destroying it, along with the contents. If you look at the side of the box, however, you will get some indication as to which amulet goes into which slot."

Pei Ke looked at one side of the box and then another until he had studied all four sides of the metal box. Wei Ken De and Mei Li did the same. Pei Ke then looked at the amulets and it became apparent to him which amulet would fit into its designated slot.

"Master, based on what I see on the box and the arrangement of the Chinese characters on the amulet, this amulet goes into this slot. Am I correct?"

"Yes, slide it into the slot. It should slide in easy with little effort."

Pei Ke lined up the amulet with the slot and slid it into the narrow opening. It slid in with almost no resistance until it reached the end of the slot, where he felt the amulet interact with the mechanism and he heard a slight metallic click. The amulet released the lever. He looked at Liu for his approval.

"Insert the other three and let's see what happens."

Pei Ke looked at each amulet to make sure he had the correct amulet for each slot. He inserted the amulets as instructed and each one released the appropriate lever.

"What do we do now?" asked Pei Ke.

"If all the amulets are in the correct location and all the levers are released, then the lid should slide open. Hold on to the box."

Pei Ke held onto the box as Liu tried to slide the lid to one side. At first, it would not move, but after a little effort, it gradually slid open, exposing the inside. There was a tray at the top of the open box. On the tray, there was a thin manuscript. Liu picked up the manuscript and opened it carefully.

After looking at it for a few moments, he carefully and with almost reverence, put it back on the tray. He lifted the tray out of the box and gave it to Pei Ke. Inside the box were many assorted manuscripts and four bars of gold.

Pei Ke realized there was a fortune in each one of the gold bars. One gold bar would make a man wealthy for the rest of his life. Four gold bars was incredible wealth. No wonder Chen had wanted to get the Liu ancestral fortune. He probably knew there was a fortune, but had no clue how vast it was.

"Master, did the Abbot have any idea what was inside of this box?"

"No, he was never told. He was only told to keep it safe. In return for keeping it safe, the temple would someday share in the rewards of being the guardian of the box. He was also led to believe, that if he took the box, there was no way he could ever benefit from it unless I or someone else within the family was aware of what was taking place. In other words stealing the box would be of no benefit to him financially."

"What are the manuscripts in the box?"

"The real fortune in this box is not the gold bars you see, but the manuscripts. The gold is real, but it is a decoy for anyone who may have gained access to the box under false pretenses. There are numerous manuscripts here. They outline the *Ancient Wisdom* and *Ancient Techniques* passed down secretly within my family for generations. There are other manuscripts covering the wisdom of the ages for better health.

"The information is an accumulation from various famous and not so famous acupuncturists and herbalists. In addition, some of the most important information has come from Buddhist and Taoist hermits who have explored the depths of human consciousness. Each of the manuscripts covers a particular aspect of good health and long life."

Liu picked up one of the manuscripts and showed it to Pei Ke. Pei Ke looked at the Chinese characters. He understood the meaning of each one of the characters, but could not understand what they meant when used together in a phrase.

"The writing is done in a scholarly fashion," said Liu. "I know you can't understand the meaning, but I can and anyone who is trained in esoteric writings of the ancients will be able to understand the message in these ancient writings.

"This first one deals with the way our ancestors combined the use of food to maximize the overall health of the body. Thousands of years ago, the ancients knew that plants had a beneficial effect on the body. Back then, humans ate the plants to enhance the wellbeing of the body. The ancient Chinese believed this information was passed on to us by the gods, and also by our trial and error in sampling the plants. The ancients found that not only were the plants helping to maintain our health, but also that certain combinations really tasted good.

"Over generations the real reason for eating these foods lost some of its meaning and people ate them because they liked the way they tasted and not because of the beneficial effect they would have on the body. Certain foods are better for us during certain seasons of the year. The energy would change during the seasons, especially from autumn to winter when our bodies have to make a major adjustment.

"This information is priceless to the right person. Imagine knowing that eating the correct food would substantially prolong your life. Some of this knowledge is still available, but not to the scope that it is represented in this manuscript. Do you remember when we were at the inn, when we first started our journey together? Mr. Yang mentioned the combinations of food, especially the use of foods that blended together because of the color of the food."

"Yes, Master, I remember."

"This manuscript covers the plants that are important in prolonging our life. If one was to adhere to what is available here, they would be able to live to a remarkably long and healthy life."

"Master, do you follow the information that is in this manuscript?"

"Yes, as much as possible, I adhere to the basic principles outlined here. There are times when it is not possible for me to adhere to the correct eating and use of herbs, but my indiscretions are few and far between. It almost always happens when I eat out away from where I can have the food prepared the way it should be prepared."

"Master, what are the other manuscripts and how do they relate to prolonged life?"

"Along with the food we eat, there are many herbs nature has provided to us. Even though the herbs are not daily food, they protect us when there is an imbalance in our energy system. This is especially important if we get sick, and when we transition from one stage of life to another. Do you remember when I told you that our life moves in cycles? Women have a seven-year cycle and men have an eight-year cycle."

"Yes, Master, I remember you telling me."

Pei Ke thought for a few seconds about all that he had learned over the last couple of years he'd been with Liu. At first, the learning was slow, but now it had been accelerated. He was thankful for the opportunity to study with Liu.

Liu went on to explain the importance of some of the other manuscripts in the metal box. As Pei Ke, Wei Ken De, and Mei Li listened to the words of their Master they realized that what he had told them was true. The true wealth in the box deals not with the gold, but with the manuscripts and the secrets they held about how to prolong one's life. A person's life could not only be prolonged for many years, but their life could be prolonged in a state of exceptionally good health. For a couple of hours, Liu briefly explained to the others the significance of what was in the metal box.

"Master," said Pei Ke. It is amazing what your family has accumulated. There is a wealth of information almost anyone would want to have. I can see why your family has safeguarded the information.

"I presume the four amulets were given to four different individuals so they could one day either continue to safeguard the information and the gold or distribute it amongst themselves."

"Yes," said Liu.

The information was kept secret with the intention of passing it on only within the family or those deemed worthy of receiving the gold and the information."

"Master, there are inscriptions on the front and back of each amulet. What is the significance of the inscriptions and characters?"

Liu pulled the amulets out of the box and laid them on the floor.

"If you look at one side you will see the Yin Yang symbol, the Five Elements of Metal, Water, Wood, Fire, and Earth. There are also the eight representations of Pa Kua. The Yin Yang, Five Elements, and Pa Kua represent the three internal martial arts of Tai Chi Chuan, Hsing-Yi Chuan, and Pa Kua Chang.

"Each one of these arts will prolong your life and build your internal energy. Each does it in a specific way. So if you learn one of these and practice it you will live longer; but if you learn all three, you will build your energy in three different ways and you should live even longer and without the many ailments most people have in life. Thus, the secret on one side of the coin is to learn the three internal Chinese martial arts and to practice them religiously."

Liu pointed to the amulets and arranged them in the appropriate sequence so they could see what he meant.

"Master, what about the other side?"

Liu turned the amulets over, arranging them again in the proper order to form a circle.

"Master," said Wei Ken De. "When the coin is separated into the four amulets, we can see there is writing on the surface of each amulet, but because of the way the coin is cut, some of the characters are shown in half and we cannot recognize the character until the amulets are put together. But even though we can now read the characters, they have no meaning for us."

"Yes, that is true, and that is why the amulets are so important, because it conveys to the four individuals, that have the amulets, that not only are the three martial arts important as seen on one side, but there are certain acupuncture points, among the hundreds of points, that will specifically help in maintaining and, if need be, restoring good health. Thus this coin is another asset for someone who wants to live a long healthy life."

"Master, the amulets, when joined together show that there are four groupings of characters. What is the meaning?" asked Mei Li."

"The first grouping is Ma Dan Yang points. Ma Dan Yang was a famous acupuncturist who believed there are twelve basic points which can be used to treat almost all healthcare issues. It isn't just the twelve points individually, but the various combinations of points that is effective. We now know these twelve points, but we do not know all the combinations he used. Acupuncturists everywhere are now experimenting with various combinations of these key points in order to enhance the value of Ma Dan Yang's findings. If you know these points, and how to use them, you will be a very effective acupuncturist.

"The second grouping is Sun Si Mao points. Sun Si Mao was another famous acupuncturist who grouped thirteen points into a category, which has come to be known as Ghost Points. Not only will these points help with basic problems, but they also have a very special therapeutic effect on our emotional stability and psyche, hence the term Ghost Points.

"The third grouping is Qi Gong points. The ancients found that there are certain acupuncture points that can open up the flow of energy when we do Qi Gong. Stimulating these points will help release any blockage along the meridian systems and allow the energy to flow, enhancing our Qi Gong experience.

"The last grouping is Long Life Points and Death Points. These are points that the ancients found and that have been passed on exclusively through my family to enhance long life. There are certain points for certain seasons, for the change of seasons, and for enhancing the flow of energy when we go through the aging process. The Death Points are acupuncture points that can be used in martial arts to either kill or severely incapacitate one's opponent.

"The grouping of points on the amulets indicates that such information exists but does not tell which points are being used. That key information is in these manuscripts. It is intended only for those who have been initiated into the Liu family as inner door students, or have been in service to the family like the servant that my brother had. For the servant and his family, it was a reward for years of faithful service."

"Master," said Pei Ke. "I am overwhelmed by the information that is here. It truly is a treasure people would actually kill for if they knew how valuable this information really is."

"Yes, that is why we keep it secret, and why my father wanted the information only to be shared with trusted individuals. Each of these identified points in these groupings is important, but the true knowledge will come from me explaining how and when to use each of these points. The amulet only reminds the person who has the amulet that this information exists. It is from my teachings that you will be able to understand the essence of what is available to you. My teachings which further explain what is on the coins are outlined on the small scrolls that are in my sack that you have been carrying for me."

The next day they all went into the village to purchase more supplies. Liu went to the temple by himself to pay respect to Kuan Yin, and while he was there, asked to see the assistant Abbot. The assistant had no word on the Abbot, and it was assumed by all that something bad had happened and that the Abbot would not be returning. As a result, the assistant was taking over as the head Abbot of the temple.

After Liu was finished paying respect to Kuan Yin, he rejoined the group, and they took their newly purchased supplies and headed north to Liu's home.

CHAPTER 63

The next morning, Liu awoke earlier than usual and walked into the main sitting area expecting not to find anyone up so early. Mei Li was there. She had made tea and was sitting in a chair, smiling.

"You are up early this morning," said Liu.

"Yes, I was waiting for you get up so I could speak with you in private."

"I see you made some tea. Let me get some and then we can talk."

Liu walked to the counter, poured himself some hot tea, and then went over to a chair opposite Mei Li and sat down. He knew what was coming and was ready for her question.

"Master Liu, I need some help."

"You know I will help you any way that I can. You and your father are family."

"As you know, I am of age for marriage. My girlfriends are getting married, and having children. I think it is time father approves of someone for me to marry or at least for me to become betrothed. I would like to get married and start a family."

"You are still young and very beautiful. You have plenty of time to get married. Why do you want to get married now?"

"There is someone I think would make a wonderful husband for me."

"Is it someone from your village area or a man related to one of your father's business associates?"

"No, it is Pei Ke."

Liu chuckled.

"Have you discussed this with your father?"

"I tried, but he is either too busy or avoids the subject."

"Why would you like to get married to Pei Ke? He has no money or any prospect of getting any. He comes from a poor family that is not very well educated and he has no business skills whatsoever."

"Master, he has what very few men have."

"What is that?"

"He is kind, loyal, honest, considerate, and you have taught him Traditional Chinese Medicine and martial arts. Besides, I think we share the same interests in life. None of the men in my village know medicine or want to practice martial arts. In addition, most of them will follow after their fathers and run around with other women or go to the brothels. I don't want that. I do not think Pei Ke would do those things."

"How do you know Pei Ke would like to marry you? Have you been so bold as to mention this to him?"

"Master, of course not. It is the custom for my father to arrange these things. I would like for you to mention this to my father."

"Are you going to talk with your father?"

"Of course, when I can get him alone, but do you have any objections to Pei Ke and me getting married?"

"It is not up to me. It is up to your father. As far as I am concerned, Pei Ke can do whatever he wants to do. He is old enough and mature enough to make his own decisions. I do know that in one of the villages we visited, some of the mothers did everything they could to entice him to return. They were looking for a husband for their daughters. That village would accept him there to practice medicine. In fact, he would be treated as a king if he were to go there."

"Is Pei Ke going to go there?"

Liu could see the apprehension in Mei Li's eyes and he almost regretted bringing up the village. She must really like him. They would make a good couple thought Liu.

"I do not know what he is going to do."

"Master, what are you going to do?"

"I am thinking about it now. I know Pei Ke would follow me wherever I went. But I also know that he would do whatever I told him to do."

Mei Li looked at Liu, not knowing what to say next. She wanted Liu to stay so she could study and learn from him as Pei Ke had been doing. She guessed Liu probably would want to continue his travels, but his ancestral home was now a responsibility he would have to address. She believed if Liu stayed, Pei Ke would also stay, unless he decided to return to that village to be with some other woman. She wondered why things had to be so difficult for her.

"Master, when do you think you will make a decision?"

"It will be some time, as I need to make decisions about this estate and Mr. Wu's estate as well. His estate has been left to my family, and since I am the only one remaining in my family, I have inherited his estate and all his lands. I will need someone to help me manage both properties and it must be someone I can trust."

Liu looked directly into Mei Li's eyes, but did not say another word. Mei Li tried to think of all the possibilities, and what they would mean for her and Pei Ke. Then she thought of her father. She did not want to leave him by himself. He had trained her to take over the family business, and he was counting on her to do so.

"Master, I guess it is not as simple as I had thought."

"Many times our emotions have a tendency to cloud the reality of what we should be doing. There are responsibilities that I have and responsibilities your father has, and there are responsibilities that you, as his daughter, have. The person who has the fewest responsibilities is Pei Ke. He can come and go as he pleases. He is fully capable of making his own decisions, and he should not feel pushed into making any particular decision. If he is forced to make a decision, which does not agree with him, he will always regret it and feel resentment towards the person or persons who forced it on him.

Do you understand?"

"Yes, Master I understand," said Mei Li.

As they were talking, a door opened and Pei Ke emerged from the hallway.

"Good morning," said Pei Ke.

Liu and Mei Li greeted him as he walked over to where the teapot was located and poured some hot tea.

"Master, how long have you been awake?" asked Pei Ke.

"Mei Li was awake when I got up and we have been talking for a few minutes."

Mei Li looked at Pei Ke, almost willing him to make something happen. She wondered what she was going to do now. There were just too many variables for her to consider. She did have to talk with her father and it had to be soon. If Pei Ke left, she would not be able to follow him. The thought of being promised to some man in her village was repulsive. She wouldn't do it. Mei Li took a chance and asked Pei Ke a question.

"Pei Ke, what are you going to do now that Teacher has resolved his problem with Chen?"

As soon as she asked the question, she wished she had not asked it. What was he going to say? Was he going to say something she didn't want to hear? She looked at Liu then back at Pei Ke.

Pei Ke was about to say something when Wei Ken De walked into the room.

"Good morning, everyone. Good morning, Teacher. Has everyone slept well?"

Everyone answered in the affirmative as he poured himself some tea. He walked over and sat down in one of the chairs.

"Master, what are we going to do today?" asked Wei Ken De.

"After we have breakfast we are going to explore the boundaries of this estate. Pei Ke has already seen some of it, and I would like for everyone to understand the extent of this land and everything it has to offer."

That day, Liu led the group through the forest, mountains, and valley, exploring the boundary lines of the Liu family estate. There were distinct markers and boulders that he pointed out to the group, and he answered their questions as they rode their horses through the land his grandfather had been awarded for his service to the emperor.

When they returned late in the day, they discussed what they had seen. The three of them were really impressed with what they saw. Each expressed why someone would want to have this land. It was a perfect place.

"Master, this land is beautiful," said Pei Ke. "You were very lucky to grow up here as a child. It is the perfect place to have a family. There is everything that anyone would ever need. There are fish in the river, fruit on the trees, and grazing land for sheep, cattle, and horses. It is a perfect place. Don't you agree Mei Li?"

Pei Ke looked at Mei Li. Her heart skipped a beat.

"Yes, it really is a beautiful place," said Mei Li.

"Yes, it would be a perfect place for a family," said Liu. "It hasn't changed in many years. The only change has been the addition of more sleeping quarters for the expansion of the family. Unfortunately, those of my family who lived here are now all gone and it is only me. In my later years, I have really missed not having a family. It would be nice to have children running around, enjoying themselves like I did."

The group talked for a couple of hours before each retired one by one for the evening. Mei Li sat there by herself. She started to cry as she thought of her desire to be married to Pei Ke. It was now almost an obsession on her part. It was unfair for her as a grown woman to want someone to share her life with and not know who it was going to be. Before she went to bed, she visualized herself and Pei Ke living on the Liu estate with happy children running around. She took this thought with her as she prayed to Kuan Yin. Finally, she fell into a deep peaceful sleep.

CHAPTER 64

The next day everyone assembled early in the morning, waiting for Liu Bin to set the course of action for the day.

"This morning I would like to pay respects to my parents and ancestors and I would like to do this alone. Please have breakfast and leave a little for me. I will be at the family graveyard for a while. When I return, we are going to ride to Mr. Wu's place and stay there for the evening. I do not remember if there are any supplies there, so be sure and bring something for us."

Without waiting for a reply, Liu walked out the door and went to the gravesite. He went from one marked grave to another. At each one of them, he read the inscription on the stone and recalled the face of the deceased as best he could. For those who had gone long before him, he imagined what they looked like. When he was done visiting with his brother and the recently deceased, he bowed to them and told them that he had upheld the honor of the family and had taken revenge for their untimely deaths. He assured them the land was still intact and Chen's false claims to the land had been dealt with appropriately. He promised that during his remaining lifetime the land would always be held in his name.

After he paid respects to his ancestors, Liu walked back to the main living area. The others had finished breakfast and were seated, drinking tea.

Liu sat down at the table and ate the food that Mei Li had placed there for him.

"Master, when will we be leaving?" asked Pei Ke. "Is there anything other than supplies that you want us to take to Mr. Wu's?"

Liu did not answer the question. He ate his food in silence as he thought of his late family. When he finished eating, he abruptly said.

"Let's go."

He stood up and walked out the door. The horses were already saddled and this pleased Liu as he climbed on his horse. The others followed his example and they rode off.

They arrived that night at Wu's place. After they had brought the supplies into the house, they sat in the main sitting area and drank hot tea.

"Master, what are we going to do here?" asked Mei Li.

"We are going to explore the compound as well as the lands. Wu had no children, and there are no remaining relatives I am aware of. In his will, Wu gave my family this house and all the lands deeded to him by the emperor. There was no mention in the will of any specific heir. It was just willed to the family, meaning it should go to the eldest member of the family. By default, I am the legal heir of this house and its lands, and I want to see the extent of the holdings."

"How do you know where the boundaries are located?" asked Pei Ke.

"Wu described the boundaries as they appeared on the deed from the emperor. He hid the information in a safe place and I was told many years ago where to look. When I came here after returning from Beijing, I went to the hiding place and read the documents that proved Wu was the rightful owner of the land. I still do not know exactly where the boundaries are located, so we are going to try to find them today. Wu did the same thing as my ancestors, and marked the boundaries so the land could be easily transferred. All we need to do is follow the directions from the documents and we should know the extent of the land. I would like all of us to do this. We will start tomorrow."

That was the clue for everyone to retire to their individual rooms for the night. Pei Ke said goodnight to everyone and went to his room. Liu followed suit and walked down the hallway to the bedroom he was going to use for the stay at Wu's. Wei Ken De was getting up from his chair when Mei Li touched his arm.

"Father, before you go to sleep, can I visit with you for a few minutes?"

"Of course," said Wei Ken De as he sat down next to Mei Li. "What is it you would like to discuss?"

"Father, I have tried to discuss a very important question with you on several occasions but there is always an interruption."

"Good there is no interruption now. What is it that is so important at this hour of the evening?"

"Father, it is time I think of my future."

"You have a good future running the business. That is why you have been included in everything I do."

"Father, you know what I'm talking about. My future husband."

"I mentioned to you before that there are a couple of nice men in the village. Do you want me to approach the families to see if there can be an arranged marriage?"

"No, never. These men you mentioned are terrible. I'll be treated as a slave and a second class person within some other home. I will have to wait on the mother-in-law for each and every one of her whims. I don't want to do that. I'll have no time to help with the business. Father, please help me."

"What is it you want?"

"I want your permission to marry Pei Ke."

He smiled fondly.

"I have already talked with teacher and we have agreed it is the best thing for both of you. However, Pei Ke does not know anything about it."

"Father! Why haven't you told me? You know I have been quite anxious about this for some time."

"Careful, Teacher has not talked with Pei Ke yet. He feels it is important for Pei Ke to make such an important decision himself. As you know, Pei Ke has been accepted into the Liu family. I think teacher will eventually talk with him about his future. You are going to have to be patient."

"Yes, father. Thank you."

CHAPTER 65

The next morning Liu took the document dealing with the boundary lines and the four of them spent the day traveling from one boundary point marker to the next. At the end of the day, they arrived back at the Wu compound.

"Master, this is almost as big as your estate," said Wei Ken De. "How are you going to manage both pieces of land, let alone each house? It would be a full time job to just manage one of these places."

"Yes, I am aware of that. Do you have any suggestions on what I should do?"

"Master, it is not my decision," said Wei Ken De.

"I know it is not your decision, but do you have any ideas," said Liu. "Do any of you have any ideas on how to manage this property?"

Liu looked at Pei Ke and Mei Li. They both shook their head. The four of them spent a few days at the Wu estate before returning to the Liu estate.

———————————

When they arrived back at Liu's ancestral home, Liu asked to be left alone for the night. The next day, he said that he was going to go into the village and would be back before sunset.

While Liu was away, they sat at the table sipping their tea. Mei Li kept looking at Pei Ke, wondering how she could convey her interest in him. Pei Ke would occasionally look at Mei Li and wondered what it would be like to be married to her. The more he thought about it, the more he was convinced it was what he wanted. The only problem was his lack of money and family prestige. This whole process of Mei Li and Pei Ke looking at each other was noticed by Wei Ken De, who shook his head and chuckled to himself.

Liu arrived back that evening and once again asked not to be disturbed. He went to his room. Unbeknownst to the rest of the group, Liu sat in his room and meditated many hours. He was looking for guidance from the Universal Energy. He needed to make some very important decisions that would affect all of them. After he finished meditating, he went to sleep. The sleep was peaceful as his mind and Universal Energy became one in unison, and he was able to make conscious and unconscious decisions appropriate for everyone involved.

CHAPTER 66

For the next two months, Liu and the others varied their stay between his ancestral home and Wu's place. Liu showed them the intricacies of how to run and manage an extended estate. During this time, they formed a very close bond, a bond that was more than just teacher and student. They worked as a team, each knowing to some extent the strengths and weaknesses of the others. Even though they worked on the two estates, Liu always took time first thing in the morning to practice martial arts, Qi Gong, or weapons with the group. Each day Pei Ke received at least two hours of advanced instruction in Traditional Chinese Medicine.

The weather turned warmer and spring was in full swing. The trees were starting to burst forth with leaves. The fruit trees in the valley started to bear their fruit. From what they could see, it would be a bountiful summer of more fruit than they could possibly eat in one year.

Mei Li asked her father a couple of times if he or Liu had spoken to Pei Ke and each time she was told to be patient. Liu made several trips into the village by himself. Wei Ken De and Mei Li made trips back to their home to make sure all was well with their family business.

During one of these trips, when Liu and Pei Ke were alone, Liu sat down with Pei Ke.

"Pei Ke, what are your plans?"

"Master, I have no plans. Whatever you are doing or going to do, is what I want to do."

"How do you like living here on this estate? It really is quite peaceful, is it not?"

"Master, it is an ideal place to live. I understand why you love it so much. It is the perfect place to bring up a family and you were very fortunate to have had this experience."

"Pei Ke, I noticed you had an attraction to Hua Yee and Mei Li. Hua Yee unfortunately is dead. I thought a couple of times marriage between you two would have been ideal. However, it is never going to happen. I do not know what your true feelings were for her, but I know she had feelings for you."

"Master, you are correct I have feelings for both Hua Yee and Mei Li. They are both beautiful and each one of them has certain extraordinary attributes, which would have been perfect for any man. But, because of my position in life, I've never thought a marriage with either one of them would be possible. The girls in the village where we stayed are more compatible with my social status."

"Wei Ken De and I have had a discussion about the future of Mei Li. We have also had a discussion about your future. It is my firm belief your martial arts ability will someday be extraordinary and your skills as a doctor will be just as extensive. However, you need to see things from a different perspective. What you have learned from me, while instructive, is very one-sided. You need to get additional experience from others.

"I and Wei Ken De feel that marriage between you and Mei Li would be appropriate."

Pei Ke stared at his teacher for a moment.

"Master, I do not know what to say. I'm lost for words. I never expected this in my wildest dreams."

"I need to make sure this union is acceptable to you. Your parents are not here, and since you have been accepted into my family, I am representing you in this union between two families. Would this marriage be acceptable to you?"

"Master, it would be the greatest honor in the world."

"Are you sure you have no hesitation because of your past feelings for Hua Yee or the flirtation from the girls in the village we stayed in."

"Master, I have learned from you that we all have to move on. Yes, marriage with Hua Yee would have been nice and, yes, I think we could have been happy, but as you said, it isn't going to happen now. A union with Mei Li would make me very happy, but does she feel the same way?"

"Wei Ken De is discussing it with her now. When they return and if Mei Li has responded, as I believe she will, there will be an agreement between him and I. We will present you two together for a matrimonial ceremony at the temple. As you know the custom is not to consult the children, but for the parents to make all the arrangements and the children to accept what is planned. In this instance, with both you and Mei Li, the circumstances are very different. Mei Li was brought up to be very independent which is different from the custom in this country for young women. With you, I am acting as your father."

"Master, I am honored to be part of your family and I will be honored to be part of Wei Ken De's family. I have the best of both situations."

"If you agree to this union, there are responsibilities that go with it. You must accept the fact she is independent and she has a business to run when her father passes away. You need to respect her for who she is."

"Yes, Master, I understand, and I accept those conditions."

"There is more but I will explain it to you when they return.

At the same time Liu Bin was discussing the marital arrangements with Pei Ke, Wei Ken De and Mei Li were having a similar discussion. Even though the two groups were miles apart, there was a feeling amongst all parties that it was the right thing to do. The details were to be discussed upon the arrival of Wei Ken De at the Liu ancestral home.

The following day, Liu went again by himself to the village. As he had done before on his other visits, he talked with the local people. These were individuals who had known the Liu family for many years. He discussed the situation about his estate, asking the elders for their advice. He spent time once more with the acting Abbot, who had assumed full responsibility for the activities of the temple and was fully integrated into the workings of the temple.

Liu ate lunch at the restaurant of his friend and inquired about the latest gossip floating around the village. The only gossip was the disappearance of the Abbot. Everyone was thankful that Chen was dead. There were many theories about what had happened to the Abbot, but no one had seen him or the monk who was with him, since the day they'd disappeared.

He returned to find Pei Ke working in the barn, repairing one of the stalls. That night Pei Ke and Liu had a long discussion about what had transpired since they first met on the mountain. Liu mentioned that an awkward young man was now becoming not only an accomplished martial artist but also a doctor. Soon, in the not too distant future, he would be out on his own and one day he would be passing the knowledge he learned on to others.

CHAPTER 67

The following evening, just before the sun started to set, Wei Ken De and Mei Li arrived. Pei Ke and Liu Bin heard them ride up to the compound and they were waiting for them as they walked in the door. It was obvious that Mei Li was very apprehensive. She looked first at Liu and then at Pei Ke, but she could not discern anything from their appearance.

"Come in," said Liu. "We have some hot tea in the pot. How was your trip?"

"It was fine," said Wei Ken De. "Did we miss anything while we were gone?"

"No," said Liu. "I am glad you two arrived when you did. It will give us time to talk."

Liu looked at Wei Ken De and noticed a slight nod from him. Liu smiled and Wei Ken De was satisfied everything was set in motion.

"Mei Li and Pei Ke this conversation deals with you both. Wei Ken De and I have had a couple of conversations concerning your future. We feel you two know each other well enough that we have agreed that according to our customs, a marriage between our two families would be good for both families. Pei Ke has been accepted into my family and is of age. Your father, Mei Li, has indicated you are of age and marriage with Pei Ke would be in the best interest of your family. Therefore, unless there is a major objection between the two families, you two are betrothed to each other as of now. Congratulations."

"Congratulations," said Wei Ken De, smiling.

Mei Li stood up and put her arms around her father.

"Thank you, father. I am so happy."

Pei Ke stood up and bowed to Wei Ken De.

"I will always take care of your daughter, and I will treat her with dignity and respect. Hopefully, we can have many children together."

Mei Li walked over to Pei Ke and bowed to him.

"Pei Ke, I will be a faithful wife to you and will always perform my wifely duties. I will always support you and will bring honor to this union. I will give you many male offspring. Father, you will have many grandchildren to play with and to spoil. Pei Ke, you and my father, can teach them martial arts."

"Mei Li, this is one of the happiest days of my life. From the moment I met you, I was sure you would be the perfect wife for me. I think we both are very lucky to be in this situation. Many other couples are destined to live their lives in ways that aren't pleasant. You and I will raise our children in the traditions of both of our families."

She sat down next to him. Wei Ken De and Liu Bin could see the happiness in their faces. The four of them talked enthusiastically for a couple of hours. At a little break in the conversation, Liu interrupted them.

"I am pleased both of you are so happy. There are many wonderful years ahead for each of you. You two will experience things Wei Ken De and I will never have the chance to experience. Treat each other with respect and you two will live long happy lives.

"You should now discuss your future. I am tired and would like to meditate. Please continue with your joyous conversation and in the morning we will rise early and practice Qi Gong."

Liu went to his room and meditated for a couple of hours and then fell asleep. Wei Ken De talked with Mei Li and his soon to be son-in-law for a while and then went to bed. Mei Li and Pei Ke stayed up and discussed the kind of things that newly engaged couples talk about.

CHAPTER 68

The next morning Liu was up early practicing Qi Gong when Wei Ken De joined him in the courtyard. Together they practiced for over an hour, until Pei Ke and then Mei Li joined them. The four of them practiced for another hour when it started to rain. They ran into the house as the rain and thunder descended on the valley. They all interpreted the rain as a sign of new beginnings.

Breakfast was composed of rice with mixed vegetables and plenty of green tea. After breakfast, Liu asked that they all sit together in the main sitting area.

He went into his room and came out with rolled up pieces of rice paper. He sat down in one of the chairs and put the pieces of rice paper on the table for everyone to see. He poured himself some tea and then looked at each one before he spoke.

"We will go into the village today and visit with the new Abbot. It is appropriate we have the proper ceremony and documentation of this union through marriage. It would be the custom to have you, Mei Li, married in your own village, but I hope that you do not mind being married here?"

Mei Li and her father looked at each other and both of them indicated verbally that they had no problem being married here.

"What about you, Pei Ke?"

"Master, whatever is agreed upon with everyone else is fine with me. Where I get married is not the important thing. The location of our marriage is not going to determine my happiness, and I don't think it's going to determine Mei Li's happiness. Whatever you three decide is fine with me."

Pei Ke looked at Mei Li and smiled. Everyone could see Mei Li was very happy and no further discussion was necessary.

"As you know, Uncle Wu had no children and no known relatives. He left his estate to the Liu family and since I am the last of the Liu family, by default the land belongs to me. I have consulted with the Abbot and the elders of the village about Wu's land and other things and have made a few decisions that I would like to share with the three of you.

"First, I am going to retain ownership of the land that has been in my family for so many years. This I promised my ancestors and I have made arrangements with some of the adjacent landowners to look after the property. They will be able to cultivate the land and harvest the fruits of their labor. They will also maintain the house and other buildings and make sure they are always clean. I have told them that you may visit the place anytime and use the main house facilities as you wish. Even though I own the land and have had the necessary information recorded at the temple, I am going to will the property to Wei Ken De. However, I am going to hold on to the deed.

"Second, I am going to do the same thing with Uncle Wu's property. The necessary information has been recorded at the temple. Again, I am going to hold onto the deed, and local land owners will look after the property and be able to cultivate the land and enjoy the fruits of their labor. You can visit the house and stay there at any time.

"Third, I would like for you, Pei Ke, to do two things. One, I have prepared a letter for you to take to Dr. Tsao at your earliest opportunity. He will, at my request, continue your education in Traditional Chinese Medicine. He is very good and has studied with others who are also capable of giving you insight into some of the more esoteric aspects of the healing arts. You should spend as much time there as necessary and I am asking Mei Li and Wei Ken De to allow you to do so.

"Fourth, I have already talked with Wei Ken De and he has agreed to continue your martial arts instruction. You and Mei Li will live and study under his guidance. You learn quickly, Pei Ke, and have already proven yourself to be an honorable, capable, and trusted student. Training under his guidance will enhance your skill level to a degree that will surprise you.

"Fifth, I am going to retain one of the gold bars. One will go to you Wei Ken De. This is the bar that should have gone to the servant's boy, but since he is dead, you may have it. One bar goes to the temple to help maintain temple activities. A second bar goes to the temple, but is to be used to help the poor or those in need.

Three of the amulets will go to you three. The fourth one is for me to keep. Remember, these amulets are key to the manuscripts. Wei Ken De is going to take all the manuscripts and keep them for me. I expect you three to commit the information on these manuscripts to memory; however, remember, they and the information they contain are not to be shared with anyone except the most trusted of individuals.

"Sixth, I have unfinished business in Beijing. After you two have been married, I will be going there to rectify a situation that needs my attention. When I leave, you three are welcome to stay here or at Mr. Wu's. Or, you can return to your own place. If so, be sure both places are closed and locked. I will give you the names of the elders and adjacent landowners of both properties who will look after the land. I encourage you to visit with them before you leave, and to always remain in contact with them. They are good people and they will go out of their way to help you."

All three looked at him dumbfounded. It was Pei Ke who ventured the question.

"Master, can we go with you?"

"No. Pei Ke you now have newly acquired responsibilities. Life keeps changing and you must change with it. Your major responsibility is to your upcoming wife. Someday you will have the responsibility of a father. You need the wisdom to understand this and to change your priorities.

"Mei Li, you are still Wei Ken De's daughter and you must honor your father and the memory of your mother, but you now must also have the wisdom to understand that you are accepting the responsibilities of a wife and someday the responsibilities of a mother. You have a very difficult balancing situation. When you are in doubt, pray to Kuan Yin and she will give you the guidance as to what to do. You can also ask the Universal Energy in my name and you will get your answer.

"Master, when will you return?" asked Mei Li.

"I will stay in Beijing for some time. I will be at the hospital. Pei Ke knows where it is located. They will know where I am and how to get in touch with me. I can't say right now when I will be returning. In my absence, just look after the lands."

———————————

Pei Ke and Mei Li's wedding was held two weeks later in the temple. It was a customary Buddhist wedding. Many in the village came to see the new bride. It was a joyous occasion. Liu Bin was happy to see Pei Ke and Mei Li so much in love. Wei Ken De was doubly happy. He had a fine son-in-law and his daughter was going to remain at home.

Shortly after the wedding, the four of them were resting in the sitting room of Liu's house. As they were sipping their tea, Liu gave an amulet to Wei Ken De, Mei Li and Pei Ke. He took the fourth piece and put it on the table, tracing its outline and all the characters on the paper. He then put the fourth amulet around his neck and gave the drawing of the fourth amulet to Wei Ken De.

"Wear these amulets around your neck at all times. I have the missing piece and will always keep it in my possession. If it is ever presented to you, then you will know that the person who presented it is a special person and should be treated with respect, for I gave it to him or her willingly and with instructions."

A couple of days later, Liu announced before going to bed that he would be leaving the following morning. He was going to leave the horses there for them to look after. He preferred to walk to Beijing. It would give him time to think. The next morning, he arose and the four of them did Qi Gong. They prayed to Kuan Yin. Liu then visited the gravesite of his ancestors and mentally told them what he was going to do. He said goodbye to Wei Ken De and Mei Li.

Pei Ke decided to walk with Liu for a while. Neither one of them spoke as they headed out the main gate. After a few minutes, Liu turned and looked back at the compound. Yes, he had spent many a good day there when he was young. It was now time to move on. In the twilight of his years, he had the wisdom to do what was right and not what was convenient. They walked together for another couple of minutes.

Liu stopped and put his arms around Pei Ke. They hugged each other tightly. Pei Ke felt Liu putting his hands on the back of his head, then on his upper back, and finally on his lower back. Pei Ke suddenly felt a warm glow being infused inside his body. It was energy he had never felt before. It was passing from Liu directly to him. It permeated first into his lungs and then into his intestines and stomach, and then throughout his body to the very core of his nature. Instantly, he knew that the Universal Energy that Liu experienced was being passed on to him. He was now the caretaker.

Tears ran down both of their cheeks. Pei Ke bowed low to his master and Liu bowed the same to him. Liu turned and walked down the road in the valley to where the road started to incline towards the peak. He never looked back as he faded into the distance. He was looking forward to where the roads split. He was going to take the path to the left. Pei Ke cried to himself as Liu disappeared from sight. He promised Liu Bin he would make him proud in all his actions and above all, he would defend the Liu estate to the best of his ability. He never saw Liu Bin again.

CHAPTER 69

A hundred miles away Chen Chang's wife and twenty-year old son were anxiously awaiting word from Chen Chang. From what he had previously told them, the land to the west had been left to them by his father, and it would soon be their new home. He was only going to be gone for a couple of months and now he was overdue.